Best of Five MCQs for the MRCP Part 1

Volume 1

T0177516

Best of Five MCQs for the MRCP Part 1

Volume 1

Edited by

Iqbal Khan

Consultant Gastroenterologist and Associate Director of Undergraduate Education,
Northampton General Hospital, Northampton, UK

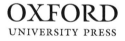

OXFORD
UNIVERSITY PRESS

OXFORD
UNIVERSITY PRESS

Great Clarendon Street, Oxford, OX2 6DP,
United Kingdom

Oxford University Press is a department of the University of Oxford.
It furthers the University's objective of excellence in research, scholarship,
and education by publishing worldwide. Oxford is a registered trade mark of
Oxford University Press in the UK and in certain other countries

Published in the United States of America by Oxford University Press
198 Madison Avenue, New York, NY 10016, United States of America

British Library Cataloguing in Publication Data

Data available

Library of Congress Control Number: 201694 122

Set ISBN 978–0–19–878792–1
Volume 1 978–0–19–874672–0
Volume 2 978–0–19–874716–1
Volume 3 978–0–19–874717–8

Printed in Great Britain by
Clays Ltd, Elcograf S.p.A.

PREFACE

The Membership of the Royal College of Physicians (MRCP) is a mandatory exam for trainees in the UK intending to enter a career in a medical speciality. The MRCP exam has three parts: MRCP Part 1 (written paper); MRCP Part 2 (written paper); and MRCP Part 2 Clinical Examination (PACES).

The MRCP (UK) Part 1 Examination is designed to assess a candidate's knowledge and understanding of the clinical sciences relevant to medical practice and of common or important disorders to a level appropriate for entry to specialist training. Candidates must sit two papers, each of which is three hours in duration and contains 100 multiple choice questions in 'best of five' format. These are designed to test candidates' core knowledge, the ability to interpret information, and clinical problem solving. The MRCP Part 1 requires a huge breadth of information to be revised.

Whilst books and resources are available, there is a huge variation in the number and quality of practice questions available. Online revision websites can be very expensive and impractical for busy junior doctors in clinical posts. These three volumes have been written with these busy junior doctors in mind and are designed to be studied one volume at a time. The three volumes together cover the full syllabus of the MRCP part 1 exam, and the number of questions per speciality is proportional to that seen in the exam. It is suggested that doctors preparing for the exam should carry one of the books into work each day and use every opportunity to study, even if it is for brief intervals. When time permits a more detailed review of the subject should take place to ensure full understanding of each topic.

The questions have been written and reviewed by experts in their respective fields and I would like to use this opportunity to thank each and every one of them for their excellent contributions.

Iqbal Khan

ACKNOWLEDGEMENTS

A small selection of questions have been kindly reproduced from *Oxford Assess and Progress: Medical Sciences*, edited by Jane Chow and John Patterson, with series Editors Kathy Boursicot and David Sales, © Oxford University Press 2012.

CONTENTS

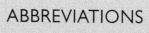

ABBREVIATIONS

µmol/L	micromoles per litre
A&E	Accident and Emergency
ABG	arterial blood gas
ABPM	ambulatory blood pressure monitoring
ACE	angiotensin-converting enzyme
ACEI	angiotensin converting enzyme inhibitor
AF	atrial fibrillation
AICD	automatic implantable cardioverter defibrillators
AIT	amiodarone-induced thyroiditis
ALT	alanine aminotransferase
AML	acute myeloid leukemia
AMP	adenosine monophosphate
ANCA	antineutrophil cytoplasmic antibodies
ARB	angiotensin II receptor blocker
ARVC	arrhythmogenic right ventricular cardiomyopathy
ASD	atrial septal defects
ATP	adenosine triphosphate
AV	atrioventricular
AVSD	atrioventricular septation defect
BD	bis in die
BLA	biological licence application
BMD	bone mineral density
BMI	body mass index
BNF	British National Formulary
BP	blood pressure
bpm	beats per minute
Ca_2	calcium
CABG	coronary artery bypass graft
CAD	coronary artery disease

cAMP	adenosine 3′,5′-cyclic monophosphate (cyclic AMP)
CF	cystic fibrosis
CGG	cytosine-guanine-guanine
CHF	congestive heart failure
CpG	cytosine-phosphate-guanosine
Cl	chlorine
CK	creatine kinase
CLL	chronic lymphocytic leukemia
CML	chronic myelogenous leukemia
CMR	cardiac magnetic resonance
CMV	cytomegalovirus
CO_2	carbon dioxide
COMT	catechol-O-methyltransferase
COPD	chronic obstructive pulmonary disease
COX	cyclo-oxygenase
CPVT	catecholaminergic polymorphic ventricular tachycardia
Cr	creatinine
CRP	C-Reactive Protein
CSF	cerebrospinal fluid
CT	computed tomography
CTA	clinical trial application
CTPA	CT pulmonary angiography
CTLA4	cytotoxic T-lymphocyte antigen 4
CXR	chest X-ray
DDR	discoidin domain receptor
DEXA	dual energy X-ray absorptiometry
DLBCL	diffuse large B-cell lymphoma
DMPS	dimercaptopropanesulphonate
DPG	diphosphoglycerate
DVT	deep vein thrombosis
DZ	dizygotic
EBV	Epstein–Barr virus
ECG	electrocardiogram
EDTA	Ethylenediaminetetraacetic acid
EGFR	epidermal growth factor receptor.
ELISA	Enzyme-linked immunosorbent assay

EMG	electromyogram
ESR	erythrocyte sedimentation rate
FAP	familial adenomatous polyposis
FBC	full blood count
Fc	fragment crystallizable
FEV	forced expiratory volume
FFP	fresh frozen plasma
FNA	fine-needle aspiration
FVC	forced vital capacity
GCS	Glasgow Coma Scale
g/dL	grammes per decilitre
GI	gastrointestinal
GTN	glycerol trinitrate
GP	general practitioner
GPBB	glucose phosphate isoenzyme BB
Hb	haemoglobin
hCG	human chorionic gonadotropin
HCM	hypertophic cardiomyopathy
HCO_3	bicarbonate
HDL	high-density lipoprotein
HDU	high dependency unit
HER	human epidermal growth factor
HLA	human leukocyte antigen
HMG	human menopausal gonadotropin
HOCM	hypertrophic obstructive cardiomyopathy
ICD	implantable cardioverter defibrillator
IgD	immunoglobulin D
IFN	interferon
IgG	Immunoglobulin class G
IM	intramuscular
IND	investigational new drug
INR	international normalized ratio
ITU	intensive treatment unit
IU/ml	international units per millimetre
IV	intravenous
IVIg	intravenous immunoglobulin

JNK	Jun N-terminal kinase
K	potassium
kg	kilogram
KPa	kilo Pascal
LABA	long-acting beta agonist
LBBB	left bundle-branch block
LDH	lactate dehydrogenase
LDL	low-density lipoprotein
LFT	liver function test
LMW	low molecular weight
LMWH	low molecular weight heparin
LVEF	left ventricular ejection fraction
LVOT	left ventricular outflow tract
M	motor response
MAPK	mitogen-activated protein kinase
mcg/l	microgram per litre
MCV	mean corpuscular volume
mg	milligramme
MGUS	monoclonal gammopathy of unknown significance
MHRA	Medicines and Healthcare Products Regulatory Agency
MI	myocardial infarction
mmHg	millimetres of mercury (torr)
mmol	millimols per litre
MMR	measles–mumps–rubella
MRI	magnetic resonance imaging
ms	milliseconds
MST	morphine sulphate
MU	million units
MVA	malignant ventricular arrhythmia
MYC	myelocytomatosis viral oncogene homologue
MZ	monozygotic
NA	sodium
NDMA	N-methyl-d-aspartate
NIPPV	nasal intermittent positive pressure ventilation
NMJ	neuromuscular junction
NMR	nuclear magnetic resonance

NPH	Neutral Protamine Hagedorn
NRTI	nucleoside reverse transcriptase
NSAID	nonsteroidal anti-inflammatory drug
NSTEMI	non-ST-elevation myocardial infarction
NYHA	New York Heart Association
O_2	oxygen
od	omni die
ONJ	osteonecrosis of the jaw
$PaCO_2$	potential carbon dioxide
PAH	p-aminohippuric acid
PaO_2	potential oxygen
PASI	Psoriasis Area and Severity Index
PCI	percutaneous coronary intervention
PCOS	polycystic ovary syndrome
PCSK9	proprotein convertase subtilisin kexin 9
PDGFR	platelet derived growth factor receptor
PEG	percutaneous endoscopic gastrostomy
PET	positron emission tomography
pH	potential hydrogen
PLT	primed lymphocyte test
pO_2	potential oxygen
PNA	purine nucleoside analogue
PPAR	peroxisome proliferator-activated receptor
PSA	prostate specific antigen
PT	prothrombin time
PTT	Partial thromboplastin time
PVE	premature ventricular event
RCP	Royal College of Physicians
RNA	ribonucleic acid
SAE	significant adverse event
SAH	subarachnoid haemorrhage
SC	subcutaneous
SCF	stem cell factor
SLE	systemic lupus erythematosus
SMR	sub-mucosal resection
SSRI	selective serotonin reuptake inhibitor

ST	sinus tachycardia
STEMI	ST-elevation myocardial infarction
TB	tuberculosis
TENS	transcutaneous electrical nerve stimulation
TIA	transient ischemic attack
TLK	tyrosine kinase
TMPT	thiopurine s-methyl transferase
TNF	tumour necrosis factor
TOE	trans-oesophageal echocardiography
TPMT	thiopurine methyltransferase
TRALI	transfusion-associated lung injury
TSH	thyroid stimulating hormone
TTE	trans-thoracic echocardiography
tTG	anti-tissue tranglutaminase
U&E	urea and electrolytes
U/l	units per litre
VAP	ventilator-associated pneumonia
VEGFR	vascular endothelial growth factor receptor
VSD	ventricular septal defect
VT	ventricular tachycardia
VTE	venous thromboembolism
WBC	white blood cell count
WCC	white cell count

1. **Which of these could cause a reduced transfer factor?**
   A. Left-to-right shunt
   B. Exercise
   C. Convalescent asthma
   D. Pulmonary haemorrhage
   E. Emphysema

2. **Hemispatial neglect is usually associated with lesions to which region of the brain?**
   A. Right parietal lobewe
   B. Left parietal lobe
   C. Left temporal lobe
   D. Both occipital lobes
   E. Right frontal lobe

3. **A couple with a 3-year-old daughter who has Turner syndrome have come to the paediatric clinic. They want to discuss their daughter's prognosis with respect to both fertility and likely morbidity during the course of her life. Which of the following represents the commonest cause of death in individuals with Turner syndrome?**
   A. Aortic aneurysm rupture
   B. Gynaecological malignancy
   C. Adrenal insufficiency
   D. Inflammatory colitis
   E. Ischaemic stroke

4. **With regard to lung function testing, which of the following is most likely to cause an increased transfer factor?**

    A. Pulmonary fibrosis
    B. Exercise
    C. Acute asthma
    D. Pulmonary oedema
    E. Emphysema

5. **You review a 22-year-old man who complains of a lump in his scrotum. He says it is painful and has been slowly increasing in size over the past 6–9 months. On examination he has a left testicular mass. You wonder if he may have a seminoma. Which of the following tumour markers is likely to be raised?**

    A. HER-2
    B. CA-19-9
    C. Placental alkaline phosphatase
    D. CA 27-29
    E. CA 15-3

6. **A 43-year-old landscape gardener complains of increasing shortness of breath. His pulmonary function tests show a low FEV_1 and normal gas transfer factor. Which is the most likely diagnosis?**

    A. Pulmonary embolism
    B. Sarcoidosis
    C. Pulmonary fibrosis
    D. Asthma
    E. COPD

7. **What is the main function of the mitochondria?**

    A. Package molecules into vesicles.
    B. Produce ATP as cell energy source.
    C. Bacterial phagocytosis.
    D. Regulate cell reproduction.
    E. Protein synthesis.

8. **You are taking a family history in clinic, and the patient reports a few conditions that he thinks may have occurred in his relatives. Which of the following conditions is inherited in an autosomal recessive manner?**

    A. Stickler syndrome
    B. Haemochromatosis
    C. Duchenne muscular dystrophy
    D. Tuberous sclerosis
    E. Classical autism

9. What is the mechanism of action of abatacept?

A. Anti-CD 20 antibody

B. Anti-CD 22 antibody

C. Anti-cytotoxic T-lymphocyte antigen 4 (CTLA4) antibody

D. Cytotoxic T-lymphocyte antigen 4 (CTLA4) homologue

E. Anti-TNF alpha antibody

10. You carry out a blood gas on a patient who has just been admitted to the medical admissions unit. These are the results (the patient is on room air): pH 7.28, pCO_2 = 3.0 kPa, pO_2 = 12 kPa, HCO_3 = 18 mmol/l. Which of the following causes is most likely?

A. Acute infective diarrhoea e.g. cholera

B. Chronic obstructive pulmonary disease

C. Vomiting

D. Low potassium

E. Respiratory muscle weakness e.g. myasthenia gravis

11. Which of the following conditions shows autosomal recessive inheritance?

A. Huntington disease

B. Neurofibromatosis type 1

C. Myotonic dystrophy

D. Congenital adrenal hyperplasia

E. Duchenne muscular dystrophy

12. A couple come to see you for advice, as they would like to start a family. The woman has cystic fibrosis and the man does not. He is a healthy Caucasian, and assumed to have a 1 in 25 chance of carrying the cystic fibrosis gene. Assuming they have a child naturally, what is the chance of them having a child affected by cystic fibrosis?

A. Around zero

B. 1 in 50

C. 1 in 25

D. 1 in 10

E. They will almost certainly have an affected child

13. The following is true of Pseudomonas aeruginosa:

A. It cannot cause infection in the immunocompetent

B. It is a cause of respiratory infection in the immunocompromised host

C. It is a commensal of the human gastrointestinal tract.

D. It is a Gram-positive rod

E. It is usually susceptible to co-amoxiclav

14. The following statements are all true of Penicillin except:

A. Acts by inhibiting bacterial cell wall synthesis
B. Can cause anaphylactic reactions in some patients
C. It contains a beta-lactam ring
D. Is primarily hepatically excreted
E. Is the initial treatment of choice for Group A, Beta haemolytic streptococcus infection

15. A 17-year-old girl with short stature presents with primary amenorrhoea. History taking and examination suggests a diagnosis of Turner's syndrome. Which of the following statements regarding this condition are correct?

A. Aortic valve disease is seen in 20–30% of patients
B. A shortened QT interval is a common association
C. It has no associations with autoimmune disease
D. Of sex-chromosome abnormalities, it is an uncommon cause
E. Renal abnormalities occur in <5% of patients

16. Which option correctly describes the effects of insulin action?

A. Decreased lipogenesis, and increased glycogen synthesis
B. Increased lipogenesis and decreased protein synthesis
C. Increased protein synthesis and decreased glucose transport into tissues
D. Decreased gluconeogenesis and glycogen storage
E. Decreased glycogenolysis and increased protein synthesis

17. You have been asked to test a new diuretic which is thought to have a similar mode of action to furosemide. At which site would you expect it to exert its greatest effect ion flux?

A. Collecting duct
B. Proximal convoluted tubule
C. Distal convoluted tubule
D. Descending loop of Henle
E. Ascending loop of Henle

18. Which of the following micro-organisms is Gram negative?

A. Bacillus anthracis
B. Clostridium perfringens
C. Klebsiella pneumoniae
D. Staphylococcus aureus
E. Streptococcus pneumoniae

19. **The haemoglobin dissociation curve is moved to the left by an increase in which of the following?**
    A. Temperature
    B. pH
    C. 2, 3 DPG concentration
    D. Hydrogen ion concentration
    E. Carbon dioxide concentration

20. **A 22-year-old man reports severe weight loss over several months. A CXR shows widening of the superior mediastinum, and a CT of the thorax revealed a 5 cm soft tissue mass in the anterior mediastinum. Which of these possible causes is least likely to account for the clinical picture and imaging findings?**
    A. Lymphoma
    B. Thymic tumour
    C. Germ cell tumour
    D. Thyroid carcinoma
    E. Malignant peripheral nerve cell tumour

21. **A 24-year-old man with a genetic make-up of 47 XXY attends the infertility clinic. Which one of the following is true of this genetic condition?**
    A. It is associated with an excess of facial hair
    B. It causes gynaecomastia in almost all patients
    C. It causes moderate–severe mental retardation
    D. It results in a mean adult height close to the 75th centile
    E. It presents at birth with ambiguous genitalia

22. **A 52-year-old woman is booked in for elective thyroid surgery for a large multinodular goitre. Six months after the procedure, the patient continues to complain of a hoarse voice. She is diagnosed with a (permanent) recurrent laryngeal nerve palsy. Which of the following statements regarding the anatomy of the recurrent laryngeal nerve is correct?**
    A. The left recurrent laryngeal originates from the vagus nerve at the level of the aortic arch
    B. The recurrent laryngeal nerve provides innervation to the cricothyroid muscle
    C. The recurrent laryngeal nerve provides only motor function to the larynx
    D. The right recurrent laryngeal nerve is longer than the left
    E. The right recurrent laryngeal nerve runs anterior to the subclavian artery

23. **A 66-year-old man was referred by the GP to the chest clinic because of long-standing dyspnoea. Recent blood tests done by his GP were: Na 127 mmol/l, K 5.5 mmol/l, Cl 87 mmol/l, HCO$_3$ 33 mmol/l, U 10.0 mmol/l. Which would be the most likely explanation?**
    A. Syndrome of inappropriate anti-diuretic hormone secretion
    B. On dual treatment with loop- and potassium-sparing diuretics
    C. On fluoxetine therapy for depressive disorder
    D. He has pseudohyponatraemia due to high serum lipid level
    E. He has psychogenic polydipsia

24. **You send blood cultures to the laboratory from a febrile patient, and Gram-positive cocci are seen on microscopy. Which of these bacteria are the most likely organisms?**
    A. Listeria
    B. Neisseria meningitidis
    C. Pseudomonas aeruginosa
    D. Staphylococcus aureus
    E. Haemophilus influenzae

25. **Programmed cell death is known as:**
    A. Apoptosis
    B. Phagocytosis
    C. Proteolysis
    D. Infarction
    E. Necrosis

26. **Which one of the following conditions with cardiac complications is not predominantly inherited in an autosomal dominant manner?**
    A. Arrhythmogenic right ventricular cardiomyopathy (ARVC)
    B. Ehlers–Danlos syndrome
    C. Friedreich's ataxia
    D. Marfan's syndrome
    E. Noonan syndrome

27. **Regarding familial cancers, which one of the following is correct?**
    A. Patients with hereditary non-polyposis colorectal cancer (Lynch syndrome) are at increased risk of cancers of the gastrointestinal tract only
    B. Li–Fraumeni syndrome is an autosomal dominant condition characterized by early onset breast cancers, sarcomas of soft tissue and bone, and a range of other malignancies
    C. In patients with breast cancer, genetic testing for mutations in the BRCA1 and BRCA2 genes should be offered to all patients with an affected pre-menopausal first-degree relative
    D. All patients with confirmed familial adenomatous polyposis (FAP) or at high risk of the disease should undergo annual colonoscopy from the age of 60
    E. Multiple endocrine neoplasia type I is characterized by tumours of the posterior pituitary, parathyroid glands, and pancreatic islet cells

28. **You are examining a new molecular tool for the treatment of inherited diseases. One of its potential targets is the CGG trinucleotide repeat in the 5' untranslated region which leads to hypermethylation of the adjacent promoter's CpG island in the *FMR-1* gene. What does this hypermethylation of *FMR-1* cause?**
    A. Transcriptional inactivation
    B. Aberrant RNA splicing
    C. Transcriptional over-activity
    D. Increased polyadenylation
    E. Increased protein glycosylation

29. **Which one of the following is true of achondroplasia?**
    A. Autosomal recessive inheritance
    B. Over 50% of cases result from new mutations
    C. Shorter trunk height is characteristic
    D. Patients are usually sterile
    E. Fifty percent of cases have subnormal intelligence

30. **The genetic defect in haemochromatosis is the result of which one of the following?**
    A. Gene amplification
    B. Translocation
    C. Point mutation
    D. Gene deletion
    E. Expansion

31. **Which HLA antigen has the greatest effect in kidney transplant rejection?**
    A. HLA–A15
    B. HLA-B27
    C. HLA-Cw5
    D. HLA-DR
    E. HLA-EA2.1

32. **A 73-year-old woman was referred to the outpatient clinic because of perseveration, an inability to spell 'WORLD' backwards or to interpret proverbs. Which region of the brain is most likely to be responsible for this deficit?**
    A. Dominant parietal lobes
    B. Frontal lobe
    C. Non-dominant parietal lobe
    D. Occipital lobe
    E. Temporal lobe

33. **A 78-year-old man was admitted to hospital with a sudden onset of impaired speech fluency, comprehension, and calculation. A clinical diagnosis of stroke was made. Which region of the brain is most likely to have been affected?**

   A. Dominant hemisphere
   B. Frontal lobe
   C. Non-dominant hemisphere
   D. Occipital lobe
   E. Temporal lobe

34. **A 40-year-old man with end-stage renal failure was admitted to hospital for cadaveric renal transplant. During surgery the kidney fails to revascularize properly and the surgeon suspects hyperacute rejection. Unfortunately the kidney has to be removed. Subsequent tests confirm that it has been subject to hyperacute rejection. Which antibody type is most likely to be responsible for this form of organ rejection?**

   A. Anti-CD3
   B. Anti-CD20
   C. Anti-Cw5
   D. Anti-B5
   E. Anti-DR4

35. **A 19-year-old woman was admitted to the emergency unit with a deteriorating level of consiousness. Investigations: Blood gas analysis: pH 7.26, bicarbonate 17 mmol/l, PaO_2 14 kPa, $PaCO_2$ 3.4 kPa. Blood chemistry: sodium 140 mmol/L, potassium 5.5 mmol/L, chloride 98 mmol/L, creatinine 140 micromol/L, urea of 8 mmol/L. What is the most likely cause of this patient's condition?**

   A. Acetazolamide therapy
   B. Aspirin overdose
   C. Hyperventilation
   D. Persistent vomiting
   E. Renal tubular acidosis type II

36. **A 74-year-old man was admitted to the emergency department with nausea and lethargy. He had a past medical history, including hypertension and ischaemic heart disease, and reported recent gastroenteritis. His medication included ramipril and furosemide. On examination his pulse was 95 bpm with a blood pressure of 115/72 mmHg. He had no signs of cardiac failure. Investigations: Haematology: Hb 13.6 g/dL (13.0–18.0). WCC 9.1x109/L (4–11). PLT 205x109/L (150–400). Biochemistry: sodium 142 mmol/L (137–144), potassium 7.0 mmol/L (3.5–4.9), creatinine 245 µmol/L (60–110). ECG—sinus rhythm 95 bpm, QRS duration 160 ms (80–120). What is the most important next therapy?**

    A. Intravenous calcium gluconate
    B. Intravenous insulin and dextrose
    C. Intravenous salbutamol
    D. Nebulized salbutamol
    E. Oral calcium resonium

37. **A 56-year-old woman attended for annual blood monitoring. She had a past history of type 2 diabetes and hyperlipidaemia The blood sample withdrawn produced white, opaque supernatant serum sample. What is the most likely explanation for this appearance?**

    A. Cryoglobulinemia
    B. Hypercholestrolaemia
    C. Hypergammaglobulinaemia
    D. Hyperglycaemia
    E. Hypertriglyceridaemia

38. **A 46-year-old man was reviewed in clinic because of refractory Crohn's disease. His disease was poorly controlled on oral steroids and a decision to start azathioprine therapy was made. The treating clinician elected to test thiopurine s-methyl transferase (TMPT) activity. What is the significance of low TMPT activity in this situation?**

    A. Accumulation of 6-mercaptopurine due to reduced hepatic metabolism
    B. Accumulation of 6-mercaptopurine due to reduced renal excretion
    C. Accumulation of azathioprine due to reduced hepatic metabolism
    D. Accumulation of azathioprine due to reduced renal excretion
    E. Reduced absorption of azathioprine from the gut

39. A 17-year-old girl presents to the emergency department with a second episode of angioedema in the past 6 months. There is no urticaria although she has significant oedema, stridor, and hypotension. Which of the following is most likely to be reduced during an attack?

A. C3
B. C4
C. C5
D. C7
E. C9

40. A 42-year-old man has presented to the clinic with a new diagnosis of Type 2 diabetes. He is grossly overweight with a BMI of 37. He approaches you for dietary advice. Which of the following foods contains the highest calorie load per gram?

A. Spaghetti
B. Parmesan cheese
C. Chicken breast
D. Brown sugar
E. Brown rice

41. A 45-year-old man was seen by his GP because of persistent tiredness. A series of investigations including full blood count, urea and electrolytes, liver function tests, and thyroid function tests were within normal limits apart from a potassium of 6.4 mmol/L (3.5–4.9). What is the most likely explanation for this result?

A. Adrenal insufficiency
B. Hypothyroidism
C. Red cell fragility disorder
D. Renal tubular acidosis
E. Sample haemolysis

42. You have been asked to investigate the effect of a new agent for treating diabetes on the production of branched chain amino acids. What is the best way to measure as yet unknown metabolites?

A. ELISA
B. Mass spectrometry
C. Nuclear magentic resonance spectroscopy
D. Radio-immuno assay
E. Urinary crystallization

43. **A 25-year-old woman was seen with her partner in the genetics clinic. She wishes to start a family and wants to discuss inheritance of a mitochondrial disorder which occurs in her family and leads to a range of neurological symptoms. What is the best description of the likely pattern of inheritance?**
    A. Autosomal dominant
    B. Autosomal recessive
    C. Maternal inheritance
    D. X-linked dominant
    E. X-linked recessive

44. **You have been investigating a new agent which acts via the PCSK9 pathway, which may have positive effects on the cardiovascular risk profile. What is the best description of the function of PCSK9?**
    A. Binds to the HDL receptor
    B. Binds to the LDL receptor
    C. Induces HDL synthesis
    D. Induces LDL synthesis
    E. Reduces triglyceride absorption

45. **In reference for sample size for comparative studies, which of the following best describes a type II error?**
    A. It is a false negative
    B. It fails to reject a true null hypothesis
    C. It is a false positive
    D. It shows no difference in the target populations when there is a significant difference
    E. It shows a difference in the target populations when there is not

46. **A study was carried out in which the weights of a large group of patients were measured. One patient's weight fell on the 75th centile. Which of the following best describes what this means**
    A. 75% of patients weigh more than this patient
    B. 75% of patients weigh less than this patient
    C. The patient weighs 75 kg
    D. There is a 75% chance that this patient weight is higher than other patients in the study group
    E. If the patients were charted periodically, this patient would fall into position 75

47. A study measures the haemoglobin (Hb) value for a group of patients. The standard deviation is found to be 2 g/dL and it is concluded that the data has a normal distribution. Which of the following statements is true when a normal distribution is assumed?

A. 99% of subjects are within 3 standard deviations of the mean
B. 92% of patients are within 2 standard deviations
C. 62% are within 1 standard deviation
D. M Scores can be used instead of standard deviations
E. Standard deviation is the square root of variance

48. A novel drug treatment has been developed to treat patients with epilepsy. Initial studies have been carried out on healthy volunteers and a small group of well-controlled epileptics. Which of the following is the best option for the manufacturers to get further data on this drug with a view to putting it in the marketplace?

A. Cross-sectional study
B. Double blind parallel group randomized control trial
C. Open label crossover study
D. Prospective cohort study
E. Double blind crossover randomized control trial

49. There is a general consensus that performing an endoscopic procedure on a patient without sedation causes distress. To test this further you carry out a study where you measure a group of patients' blood pressures (as a surrogate marker for distress) before and after a diagnostic gastroscopy. Which of the following tests would you use to prove that the endoscopic investigation results in a change of blood pressure and hence is likely to cause distress?

A. Paired T-Test
B. Independent T-Test
C. Mann–Whitney U test
D. Wilcoxson Rank Sum Test
E. Chi Square Test

50. Which of the following best describes standard deviation?

A. Spread of data around the median value
B. Spread of data around the mode value
C. Spread of data around the midi value
D. Spread of data around the mean value
E. Spread of data around the maximum value

51. **As a researcher, which of the following sort of studies is likely to provide you with the best evidence?**

A. Case study

B. Case-control study

C. Randomized control study

D. Cohort study

E. Meta-analysis

52. **A gastroenterology study is carried out looking at the efficacy of various treatments for varices. The modalities of treatment under investigation were the use of banding plus sclerotherapy versus banding plus a placebo injection for oesophageal varices. What type of statistical analysis should be carried out?**

A. Chi-Square test

B. Mann–Whitney U test

C. Wilcoxson Signed Rank Test

D. Paired T test

E. Unpaired T test

53. **A study is being conducted looking at the effect of ethnicity on heart rate response to a protocol driven exertion on a treadmill. Which of the following data types does ethnicity variables belong to?**

A. Ordinal data

B. Discrete data

C. Continuous data

D. Nominal data

E. None of the above

54. **Which of the following best describes an interquartile range?**

A. 25–75%

B. 25–50%

C. Middle 25% of values

D. Middle 75% of values

E. 50–75%

55. **Under defined conditions, an enzyme has a characteristic Michaelis constant, K_m, and a maximal rate of reaction, V_{max}, as shown in Figure 1.1. Which is the single defining property of the V_{max} value of an enzyme-catalysed reaction?**

A. It increases with increasing enzyme concentration

B. It decreases in the presence of a competitive inhibitor

C. It is the rate at which the substrate concentration is twice the K_m value

D. It is unchanged in the presence of a non-competitive inhibitor

E. It may have units of millimoles per litre

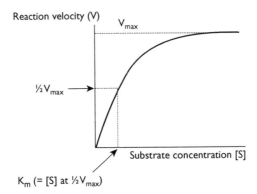

Figure 1.1 Graph. Reproduced from Chow J. & Patterson J., *Oxford Assess and Progress: Medical Sciences*, 2012 with permission from Oxford University Press.

56. **Some medicinal drugs, for example the antibiotic penicillin, exert their effect by specifically inhibiting a target enzyme. The nature of this inhibition can be either competitive or non-competitive. Which single property of a non-competitive inhibitor of an enzymecatalysed reaction best distinguishes it from a competitive inhibitor?**

    A. It bears a structural resemblance to the substrate
    B. It binds reversibly to the active site of the enzyme
    C. It changes the K_m value of the enzyme
    D. It forms a covalent complex with the enzyme
    E. It lowers the rate of the reaction except at high substrate concentration

57. **Cholera toxin causes severe diarrhoea by binding to complex oligosaccharides of certain lipids in the plasma membrane of cells lining the lumen of the intestine. To which single type of membrane lipid does cholera toxin bind?**

    A. Cerebroside
    B. Cholesterol
    C. Ganglioside
    D. Phosphatidylinositol
    E. Sphingomyelin

58. **The plasma membrane represents a barrier to the transmission of an external signal to the cell's interior. Many structures and mechanisms have evolved to facilitate chemical and electrical communication and coordination between cells. Which single effect is the immediate consequence of acetylcholine binding to a nicotinic receptor at a neuromuscular junction?**

    A. Activation of a protein kinase
    B. Activation of gene transcription
    C. Opening of ion channels
    D. Release of Ca 2 + ions
    E. Synthesis of a second messenger

59. **Following an abnormal cervical smear which showed larger and more irregular nuclei, a 37-year-old woman has a cervical biopsy which shows hyperchromatic and pleomorphic nuclei with no inflammatory cells (see Figure 1.2). Which single type of pathological tissue alteration is shown here?**

    A. Anaplasia
    B. Dysplasia
    C. Hyperplasia
    D. Metaplasia
    E. Neoplasia

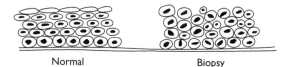

Normal   Biopsy

Figure 1.2 Normal biopsy. Reproduced from Chow J. & Patterson J., *Oxford Assess and Progress: Medical Sciences*, 2012 with permission from Oxford University Press.

60. **A 1-year-old boy developed bilateral retinoblastoma. There is a history of this tumour in his family. Genetic testing reveals a mutation in a gene on chromosome 13 called the *RB1* gene. Which single alteration of function is the most likely consequence of the mutation to chromosome 13?**

    A. Proto-oncogene activation
    B. Proto-oncogene amplification
    C. Proto-oncogene loss
    D. Tumour suppressor gene activation
    E. Tumour suppressor gene loss

61. A 25-year-old pregnant woman attends a prenatal ultrasound scan at 20 weeks. The scan shows that her fetus has a rocker-bottom foot. Which single genetic error is most likely to have caused this fetus's condition?

A. Amplification of a specific trinucleotide sequence in a gene

B. Deletion of bases within a coding region of a gene

C. Gain of one homologous chromosome

D. Loss of a portion of a chromosome

E. Point mutation of a base within a coding region of a gene

62. Leber's optic neuropathy is a genetic condition that causes blindness in young adults. When an affected woman has children, all of them inherit the disease. When an affected man has children, none of them does. Which single term describes best the mode of inheritance of Leber's optic neuropathy?

A. Autosomal dominant

B. Autosomal recessive

C. Mitochondrial

D. X-linked

E. Y-linked

63. A 78-year-old woman presents to her GP complaining of neck pain and inability to move her arm properly. Her right arm biceps and supinator tendon reflexes are absent but the triceps reflex is normal compared to her left arm. Two-point discrimination, joint position sense, and vibration and pinprick sensations are all normal. Sensory nerve conduction and electromyogram (EMG) tests reveal that the nerve conduction velocity appears normal but the compound muscle action potential size is decreased on the right. Which is the single most likely location for the underlying pathology in this patient?

A. Dorsal root

B. Neuromuscular junction

C. Peripheral nerve

D. Spinal nerve

E. Ventral root

64. Figure 1.3 is a diagrammatic representation of the spinal cord, the sympathetic chain, and the paravertebral ganglia, as well as some related structures. Which single, labelled structure in the diagram contains only unmyelinated, postganglionic sympathetic fibres?

A. Dorsal root

B. Grey ramus

C. Sympathetic chain

D. Ventral root

E. White ramus

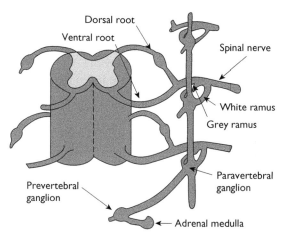

Figure 1.3 A diagrammatic representation of the spinal cord. Reproduced from Chow J. & Patterson J., *Oxford Assess and Progress: Medical Sciences*, 2012 with permission from Oxford University Press.

65. **During the production of an action potential in a nerve axon the membrane potential moves very rapidly (in about a millisecond) from close to E K, the Potassium Equilibrium Potential, to a peak just below the Sodium Equilibrium Potential, E Na. The voltage returns quickly towards the resting value, undershoots it slightly, and then returns to the resting membrane potential (Figure 1.4). Which single process must occur at the peak of the action potential before the membrane voltage can move towards E K?**

    A. Active pumping of sodium ions out of the axon
    B. Efflux of potassium out of the axon
    C. Hyperpolarization of the axon membrane
    D. Inactivation of the voltage-dependent sodium channels
    E. Influx of sodium into the axon

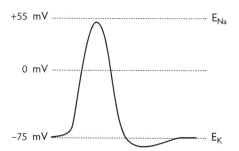

Figure 1.4 Graph. Reproduced from Chow J. & Patterson J., *Oxford Assess and Progress: Medical Sciences*, 2012 with permission from Oxford University Press.

66. **A 19-year-old man falls from his motorbike whilst not wearing a helmet. He lands on his head and loses consciousness. He is rushed to hospital where a CT scan, Figure 1.5, shows a convex-lens-shaped haemorrhage in the left temple region. Which single vascular structure is most likely to have been injured?**

    A. Cavernous sinus
    B. Middle cerebral artery
    C. Middle meningeal artery
    D. Superficial temporal artery
    E. Transverse sinus

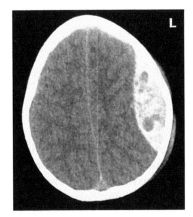

Figure 1.5 CT scan. Reproduced from Chow J. & Patterson J., *Oxford Assess and Progress: Medical Sciences*, 2012 with permission from Oxford University Press.

67. **A 20-year-old woman falls and sustains a blunt trauma to the head, but does not lose consciousness. The following day she presents to the A&E department with a severe headache. She is drowsy and starts to vomit. A computerized tomography (CT) scan of her head appears normal, but lumbar puncture shows blood in the cerebrospinal fluid. Which single condition is the most likely cause of these observations?**

    A. Cerebral venous sinus thrombosis
    B. Extradural haematoma
    C. Intracerebral haemorrhage
    D. Subarachnoid haemorrhage
    E. Subdural haematoma

68. **A 21-year-old motorcyclist has been involved in a road traffic accident. When assessed at A&E, he withdraws his arm in response to painful stimuli. He subsequently opens his eyes and moans incoherently. Which single number best describes his Glasgow Coma Scale (GCS) score?**

    A. 6
    B. 7
    C. 8
    D. 9
    E. 10

69. **A 55-year-old man suffering from Huntington's disease is unable to work out how to ride a bike. On further questioning, he correctly defines what a bike is and recollects his favourite childhood bike routes. When asked how to unlock his bike, he tells you where he keeps the padlock key. Which single type of memory is most likely to be affected in this patient?**

    A. Declarative
    B. Episodic
    C. Procedural
    D. Semantic
    E. Working

1. E. Emphysema

For MRCP Part 1, it is essential to know causes of reduced transfer factor and increased transfer factor. There are seven causes of reduced transfer factor: emphysema, acute asthma, pulmonary fibrosis, pulmonary oedema, pneumothorax, PE, and anaemia. There are six causes of increased transfer factor: pulmonary haemorrhage, left-to-right shunt, polycythaemia, early left heart failure, convalescent asthma, and exercise.

Chapman S et al., *Oxford Handbook of Respiratory Medicine*, Second Edition, Oxford University Press, 2009, Chapter 6, Diffuse lung disease, p. 36.

2. A. Right parietal lobe

This clinical sign usually arises from lesions to the right parietal lobe: in most left-dominant brains the left spacial sensory information is processed only by the right cerebral hemisphere (predominantly the parietal lobe).

Hodges JR, *Cognitive Assessment for Clinicians*, Second Edition, Oxford University Press, 2007.

3. A. Aortic aneurysm rupture

Evidence on Turner syndrome mortality comes from a cohort study from the UK which has enrolled over 3400 women with the condition. Circulatory disease accounted for 41% of excess deaths associated with Turner syndrome. Of these the SMR for aortic aneurysm was above 20, whereas for aortic valve disease it has been estimated at 17.9. Diabetes and inflammatory colitis are also more common in Turner syndrome.

Bradley-Smith G et al., *Oxford Handbook of Genetics*, Oxford University Press, Chapter 8, Chromosomes, Turner syndrome (45,X and variants).

4. B. Exercise

Transfer factor is a measure of the lungs' ability to transport oxygen into blood (and carbon dioxide out). Disease processes that limit gas transfer are therefore typically associated with reduced transfer factor, such as emphysema, acute asthma, pulmonary fibrosis, pulmonary oedema, pneumothorax, pulmonary embolus, and anaemia. Conversely, transfer factor is increased by: left-to-right shunts, polycythaemia, and exercise.

Chapman S et al., *Oxford Handbook of Respiratory Medicine*, Second Edition, Oxford University Press, 2009, Chapter 6, Diffuse lung disease, p. 36.

5. C. Placental alkaline phosphatase

CA 15-3 and 27-29 are associated with breast disease, as is HER-2. Placental alkaline phosphatase is elevated in pregnancy, seminoma, and smoking. CA 125 is raised in carcinoma of the ovary. CA 19-9 is raised in pancreatic and colorectal cancer.

Longmore M et al., *Oxford Handbook of Clinical Medicine*, Eighth Edition, Oxford University Press, 2010, Chapter 11, Oncology and palliative care, Tumour markers.

6. D. Asthma

Low FEV_1 and can give normal gas transfer factor. Acute asthma can give a reduced transfer factor whereas convalescent asthma can give an increased transfer factor.

Chapman S et al., *Oxford Handbook of Respiratory Medicine*, Second Edition, Oxford University Press, 2009, Chapter 18, Asthma.

7. B. Produce ATP as cell energy source

The mitochondria are enzyme-rich organelles that produce most of the ATP energy. Packaging and moving proteins to the outside of the cell is the function of Golgi apparatus which present as layers of membrane-covered sacs. Cell division occurs at the centriole. The ribosome contains ribonucleic acid molecules and enzymes that play roles in manufacturing proteins. Phagocytosis is the vesicular internalization of solid particles (bacteria) by immune cells. It operates at the cell membrane.

McBride HM, Neuspiel M, Wasiak S, Mitochondria: more than just a powerhouse, *Current Biology* 2006;16(14):R551–560.

8. B. Haemochromatosis

Haemochromatosis is a disorder of iron metabolism that causes iron overload and therefore complications including cardiomyopathy, liver cirrhosis, arthritis, and diabetes. Apart from a few exceptions, it is inherited in an autosomal recessive manner. Stickler syndrome is a disorder of collagen that is inherited in an autosomal dominant manner. Duchenne muscular dystrophy is a form of muscular dystrophy that is inherited in an X-linked recessive manner. Tuberous sclerosis is a disorder characterized by hamartomas in the brain, skin, and other organs. It is inherited in an autosomal dominant manner. Classical autism is not inherited in a Mendelian manner. However, there is likely to be some genetic element as the concordance rate in monozygotic (MZ) twins is much higher than dizygotic (DZ) (60–91% in MZ compared to 0–6% in DZ). There is also 45x the population risk in a sibling of an affected individual. However, the pattern of genetics is not determined and specific target genes have not been found.

Bradley-Smith G et al., *Oxford Handbook of Genetics*, Oxford University Press, Chapter 5, Common genetic conditions.

9. D. Cytotoxic T-lymphocyte antigen 4 (CTLA4) homologue

Abatacept is a cytotoxic T-lymphocyte antigen 4 (CTLA 4) homologue. It is the first in a new class of agents for the treatment of rheumatoid arthritis that selectively modulate the CD80 or CD86–CD28 costimulatory signal required for full T-cell activation. CD80 or CD86 on the surface of an antigen-presenting cell binds to CD28 on the T cell, facilitating T-cell activation. In the normal sequence of events, the naturally occurring inhibitory molecule CTLA4 is induced on the surface of the T cell. CTLA4 has a markedly greater affinity for CD80 or CD86 than does CD28, thus outcompeting CD28 for CD80 or CD86 binding. Abatacept is a recombinant fusion protein comprising the extracellular domain of human CTLA4 and a fragment of the Fc domain of human IgG1.

Genovese MC et al., Abatacept for rheumatoid arthritis refractory to tumor necrosis factor alpha inhibition, *New England Journal of Medicine* 2005;353:1114–1123. http://www.nejm.org/doi/pdf/10.1056/NEJMoa050524.

10. A. Acute infective diarrhoea, e.g. cholera

Acute diarrhoea can cause a metabolic acidosis as seen here, due to the loss of bicarbonate in the diarrhoeal fluid. The pH is low and the pCO_2 is also low. This suggests some element of respiratory compensation by hyperventilation. COPD causes a respiratory acidosis—raised pCO_2. These patients do not tend to hyperventilate so that the pCO_2 does not go down. Also, in this ABG result the pH is low and the pCO_2 is also low, so the primary problem is a metabolic acidosis Vomiting tends to cause a metabolic alkalosis due to loss of hydrogen ions from gastric secretions. Low potassium causes a metabolic alkalosis. As potassium ions move out of the cells in an effort to raise the potassium, they are exchanged for hydrogen ions which move in, causing an alkalosis. Respiratory muscle weakness e.g. myasthenia gravis causes a respiratory acidosis due to hypoventilation.

Anaesthesia MCQ website: http://www.anaesthesiamcq.com/AcidBaseBook/ABindex.php.

11. D. Congenital adrenal hyperplasia

Congenital adrenal hyperplasia shows autosomal recessive inheritance. Huntington disease, neurofibromatosis, and myotonic dystrophy are inherited as autosomal dominant traits. Duchenne muscular dystrophy is X-linked.

Tobias E et al., *Essential Medical Genetics*, Sixth Edition, Wiley-Blackwell, 2011. http://www.essentialmedgen.com/index.php.

12. B. 1 in 50

She will have two cystic fibrosis gene mutations. If he is not a carrier, then all their children will have one cf gene and one normal gene. They will therefore all be carriers and none of them will have the condition. If he is a carrier, then he will have one mutant CF gene copy (allele) and one normal copy. Their offspring would then have a 1 in 2 chance of inheriting his mutant copy and of being affected. The chance of him being a carrier is 1 in 25. Therefore the overall chance of an affected child is $1/25 \times 1/2 = 1/50$.

Tobias E et al., *Essential Medical Genetics*, Sixth Edition, Wiley-Blackwell, 2011. http://www.essentialmedgen.com/index.php.

13. B. It is a cause of respiratory infection in the immunocompromised host

Pseudomonas aeruginosa is a gram-negative rod. It is ubiquitous in the environment, particularly moist environments such as soil. It rarely causes infection in the community but can colonize sites such as chronic ulcers. It is a recognized cause of otitis externa. It can be highly pathogenic, however, particularly in immunocompromised individuals, and especially those on intensive care units, where it is a common cause of ventilator-associated pneumonia (VAP). It can cause infections of prosthetic material such as indwelling catheters. It is generally sensitive to aminoglycosides, quinolones, ticarcillin, piperacillin, ceftazidime, and carbapenems (except ertapenem); however, resistance to these agents can develop rapidly.

Torok E et al., *Oxford Handbook of Infectious Diseases and Microbiology*, First Edition, Oxford University Press, 2014, Chapter 4, Systematic microbiology, pp. 341–342.

14. D. Is primarily hepatically excreted

Penicillin is excreted by the renal tubular cells. Caution must be taken when prescribing penicillins in patients with renal failure.

Torok E et al., *Oxford Handbook of Infectious Diseases and Microbiology*, First Edition, Oxford University Press, 2014, Chapter 2, Antimicrobials, pp. 64–65.

15. A. Aortic valve disease is seen in 20–30% of patients

Turner's syndrome, first described in 1938, is the most common sex-chromosome abnormality in females affecting 1:2000 live (female) births. The condition also accounts for 15% of all spontaneous abortions with only 1/1000 embryos surviving to term. The condition is caused by complete or partial deletion of an X chromosome and the diagnosis, when suspected, is confirmed by karyotype. Prenatal diagnosis is also possible. Characteristic clinical features of the syndrome include: a webbed neck, broad chest, widely spaced nipples, and a low hairline. The most common features are short stature and primary amenorrhoea. Renal abnormalities are also common, occurring in 30–50% of patients and occasionally leading to complications such as pyelonephritis and hydronephrosis. Recognized cardiovascular abnormalities include coarctation (3–10%), aortic valve disease (20–30%), hypertension, and a prolonged QT interval. Further complications include hearing loss, hypothyroidism, and liver function abnormalities. There are recognised autoimmune associations, e.g. chronic autoimmune thyroiditis.

Turner Syndrome Support Society. http://www.tss.org.uk/.

16. E. Decreased glycogenolysis and increased protein synthesis

Insulin is a 51-amino acid peptide hormone which is synthesized by pancreatic beta cells. It is most recognized for its role in the reduction of blood glucose levels although this is only one component of its extensive metabolic profile. Glucose is liberated into the blood through the intestinal absorption of food or the breakdown of glycogen (glycogenolysis). It is also synthesized *de novo* from carbohydrate, protein, and fat precursors (gluconeogenesis). When glucose levels rise, insulin acts to promote glucose uptake, utilization, and storage, thereby reducing levels again. The uptake of glucose into adipose tissue and muscle is initiated by insulin signalling and the subsequent translocation of glucose transporters from the cytoplasm (where they are ineffective) to the plasma membrane, where they are positioned to capture glucose. Within the liver, glycogen storage is promoted through the activation of various enzymes involved in glycogen synthesis including glycogen synthase. Insulin also acts (through enzyme inhibition and further indirect actions) to reduce gluconeogenesis and glycogenolysis. The net result of these actions is a reduction in glucose levels. Insulin also has significant effects on lipid, protein, and mineral metabolism including an increase in protein synthesis and lipogenesis as well as a reduction in protein breakdown and lipolysis. These actions allow the organization of fuels for (varying) energy demands.

Tanyolac S et al., Insulin pharmacology, Types of regimens and adjustments, *Endotext*, 1st April 2008.

17. E. Ascending loop of Henle

Loop diuretics act on the sodium potassium chloride symporter which is in the ascending loop of Henle. They lead to increased excretion of chloride- and sodium-rich fluid, a fall in serum potassium and calcium, and an increase in serum bicarbonate. The proportion of sodium and water lost is greater than that lost with respect to thiazide diuretics, such that the main indication for loop diuretics is in the treatment of fluid overload.

Furosemide prescribing information, http://www.medicines.org.uk/emc/medicine/24496.

18. C. Klebsiella pneumoniae

Gram-stain appearance is often the first piece of information to emerge from the microbiology laboratory as the diagnosis is reached in a case of sepsis. It immediately allows targeting of antimicrobial therapy towards the likely cause. Common Gram-stain appearances are outlined in Table 1.1.

Table 1.1 Gram-stain appearances of common micro-organisms

Gram-positive cocci	Gram-negative cocci
Any staphylococcus species including: *Staphylococcus aureus* Any streptococcus species including: *Streptococcus pyogenes* *Streptococcus viridans* *Streptococcus pneumoniae*	*Neisseria sp. (meningitides and gonorrhoea)*
Gram-positive rods	**Gram-negative rods**
Clostridium sp. (botulinum, tetani, etc) *Bacillus anthracis* *Listeria monocytogenes*	*Escherichia coli* *Klebsiella pneumonia* *Pseudomonas aeruginosa* *Haemophilus influenza* *Legionella pneumophila*

Longmore M et al., *Oxford Handbook of Clinical Medicine*, Eighth Edition, Oxford University Press, 2010, Chapter 9, Infectious diseases, miscellaneous gram-positive bacteria.

19. B. pH

Increasing temperature, 2,3 DPG, hydrogen ions or CO? will cause the haemoglobin dissociation curve to shift to the right. An increase in PH causes a shift to the left.

Chapman S et al., *Oxford Handbook of Respiratory Medicine*, Second Edition, Oxford University Press, 2009, Appendix 1: Blood gases and acid–base balance, Conversion between arterial oxygen saturation and oxygen tension, p. 802.

20. E. Malignant peripheral nerve cell tumour

This history and CT findings are highly suggestive of malignancy. In this age group, lymphoma is the most likely cause, with thyroid carcinoma, germ cell tumours (teratoma), and thymic tumours rare but possible aetiologies. A malignant peripheral nerve cell tumour is also rare, but would be centred in the posterior mediastinum.

Chapman S, Nakielny R, *Aids to Radiological Differential Diagnosis*, Fourth Edition, Saunders, 2003, Respiratory tract, p. 185.

21. D. It results in a mean adult height close to the 75th centile

This man has Klinefelter syndrome. Patients have scant body hair and little facial hair growth. About 40% develop gynaecomastia. Klinefelter syndrome generally does not cause significant mental retardation.

Tobias E et al., *Essential Medical Genetics*, Sixth Edition, Wiley-Blackwell, 2011. http://www.essentialmedgen.com.

22. A. The left recurrent laryngeal originates from the vagus nerve at the level of the aortic arch

Due to its close proximity to the gland, the recurrent laryngeal nerve is vulnerable to damage during thyroid surgery. The nerve provides both sensory and motor function to the larynx but does not supply the cricothyroid muscle which is the only laryngeal muscle to be supplied by the superior laryngeal nerve (external branch). The left recurrent laryngeal nerve originates from the vagus nerve at the level of the aortic arch. It passes posterior to the aorta at the ligamentum arteriosum and then courses superiorly over the left main bronchus to ascend into the tracheoesophageal groove and enter the larynx inferior to the cricothyroid muscle. The right recurrent laryngeal nerve originates from the right vagus nerve and curves posteriorly around the subclavian artery before taking a more transverse course. The left recurrent laryngeal nerve has a longer course than the right.

Endocrinesurgeon.co.uk. http://www.endocrinesurgeon.co.uk/index.php/ mr-john-lynn-endocrine-surgeon.

23. B. On dual treatment with loop- and potassium-sparing diuretics

This patient has cardiac failure causing his chronic dyspnoea. Common biochemical findings of a patient on loop- and potassium-sparing diuretics would include hyponatraemia, hyperkalaemia, alkalosis, and mild dehydration. Addison's disease can produce the same biochemical picture but it does not explain his chronic dyspnoea and it is not one of the options.

Longmore M et al., *Oxford Handbook of Clinical Medicine*, Eighth Edition, Oxford University Press, 2010, Chapter 15, Clinical chemistry, hyponatraemia, p. 686.

24. D. *Staphylococcus aureus*

S. aureus is the only Gram-positive coccus in this list, and is a common cause of bacteraemia. It is important to differentiate methicillin-sensitive and methicillin-resistant *S. aureus* in patients with *S. aureus* in their blood cultures, as it is vital to give them effective treatment. The other important group of Gram-positive cocci are the streptococci. Here are the microscopic appearances of the other bacteria in the list of options: (a) *Listeria*—an aerobic Gram-positive rod; (b) *Neisseria meningitidis*—Gram-negative coccus; (c) *Pseudomonas aeruginosa*—Gram-negative rod; (d) *Staphylococcus aureus*—Gram-positive coccus; (e) *Haemophilus influenzae*—Gram-negative rod.

Torok E et al., *Oxford Handbook of Infectious Diseases and Microbiology*, Oxford University Press, Chapter 4, Systematic microbiology, Overview of Gram-positive cocci.

25. A. Apoptosis

Apoptosis is known as 'programmed cell death', which occurs with no inflammatory reaction, as opposed to necrosis which causes a local inflammatory response. Necrosis is the pathological death of one or more cells or a portion of tissue or organ. Infarction is sudden insufficiency of arterial or venous blood supply causing a macroscopic area of necrosis. Phagocytosis is the process of ingestion and digestion of solid substances by cells. Proteolysis is the decomposition of protein, primarily via the hydrolysis of peptide bonds, both enzymatically and non-enzymatically.

Alberts K et al., *Molecular Biology of the Cell*, Fifth Edition, Garland Science, 2008, Chapter 18, Apoptosis: programmed cell death eliminates unwanted cells, p. 1115.

26. C. Friedreich's ataxia

Friedreich's ataxia is inherited in an autosomal recessive fashion. This condition is associated with a cardiomyopathy and affected individuals should be screened for this complication. All of the remaining conditions are inherited predominantly in an autosomal dominant fashion, although *de novo* mutations are common. Ehlers–Danlos syndrome is associated in some cases with aortic syndromes. Noonan syndrome can be associated with pulmonary stenosis and hypertrophic cardiomyopathy. Marfan syndrome is associated with mitral valve prolapse, aortic syndromes, and aortic regurgitation.

Alper G, Narayanan V, Friedreich's ataxia, *Pediatric Neurology* 2003;28(5):335–341.

27. B. Li-Fraumeni syndrome is an autosomal dominant condition characterized by early-onset breast cancers, sarcomas of soft tissue and bone, and a range of other malignancies

Lynch syndrome (hereditary non-polyposis colorectal cancer) is associated with an increased incidence of multiple malignancies, particularly colon cancer as well as tumours of the endometrium and, less commonly, the ovary. Li–Fraumeni syndrome is an autosomal dominant condition characterized by young-onset breast cancers, sarcomas of soft tissue and bone, and a range of other malignancies including leukaemias and brain tumours. In the majority of families a germline mutation in the tumour-suppressor *p53* gene is the cause. Breast cancer is a common cancer. Up to a third of patients will have at least one relative who has also been affected with the disease, yet only a small proportion of affected patients (5–10%) will have a 'hereditary' cancer, some of which are due to mutation of either *BRCA1* or *BRCA2*. Certain features of the family history are particularly suggestive of hereditary breast cancer, including multiple relatives with breast and/or ovarian cancer, particularly if developed at <50 years of age, bilateral breast cancer or breast cancer plus ovarian cancer, and affected male relatives. NICE has issued guidelines on risk stratification and subsequent referral to screening or genetics services. Familial adenomatous polyposis is an autosomal dominant disease. A truncating mutation in the *APC* gene can be identified in up to 90% of cases. Classic FAP is characterized by the presence of >100 colorectal adenomas. Ninety percent of these patients will develop colonic cancer by the age of 45 years unless treated, as well as being at greater risk of some extra-colonic cancers, including duodenal tumours. Regular flexible sigmoidoscopy is usually offered to high-risk relatives of patients from their teens onwards with annual colonoscopies once polyps have been detected, until colonic resection is carried out. In patients with a confirmed gene mutation or presenting clinical features suggestive of the disease, surgery is the preferred management. Multiple endocrine neoplasia type 1 (MEN1) is an autosomal dominant condition characterized by a predisposition to tumours of the parathyroid glands and pancreatic islet cells, as well as tumours of the anterior pituitary. Patients are also at greater risk of other tumours, including benign tumours of the adrenal glands and carcinoid tumours.

NICE Guidelines, Familial breast cancer. http://www.nice.org.uk/nicemedia/pdf/CG41NICEguidance.pdf.

28. A. Transcriptional inactivation

Unchecked methylation of the *FMR-1* gene leads to fragile-X, a syndrome which involves developmental delay, hyperactivity, and inappropriate behaviour. Hypermethylation of the promoter of the gene causes transcriptional inactivation and is associated with an average IQ of 41. Autistic features are common. Symptoms consistent with the syndrome worsen with successive generations, a feature of some genetic disorders in which there are trinucleotide repeats.

Bradley-Smith G et al., *Oxford Handbook of Genetics*, Oxford University Press, 2009, Chapter 5, Common genetic conditions, Fragile X syndrome (FRAX).

29. B. Over 50% of cases result from new mutations

Achondroplasia is inherited as an autosomal dominant trait. Approximately 80% of cases are new mutations, the mutation is in the *FGFR3* gene, and it affects endochondral ossification. The individual is short in stature with rhizomelic (i.e. proximal) shortening of upper and lower limbs but the trunk is of relatively normal length. Complications include hydrocephalus and spinal cord/root compression. Fertility and intelligence are normal.

Horton WA et al., Achondroplasia, *Lancet* 2007;370(9582):162–172.

30. C. Point mutation

The most common genetic defect is the replacement of a cysteine amino acid with a tyrosine at position 282 (C282Y) in the *HFE* gene. The sequence of a gene can be altered in a number of ways. Gene mutations have varying effects on health depending on where they occur and whether they alter the function of essential proteins. Point mutations are substitutions, insertions, or deletions of a single nucleotide. Substitutions include: silent mutations, which code for the same amino acid; missense mutations, which code for a different amino acid; and nonsense mutations, which code for a stop and can truncate the protein. Insertions or deletions of a single nucleotide can result in a frameshift and a premature stop codon.

Wildeman M et al., Improving sequence variant descriptions in mutation databases and literature using the Mutalyzer sequence variation nomenclature checker, *Human Mutation* 2008;29(1):6–13.

31. D. HLA-DR

The UK Transplant data shows that DR mismatching has a much greater effect than that of B or A. Each antigen also appears to exert its effect at different times post-transplant, with the maximal effect of DR and B mismatching occurring within the first six months and two years post-transplant, respectively.

Overcoming Antibody Barriers to Kidney Transplant. http://discoverysedge.mayo.edu/.

32. B. Frontal lobe

These neuropsychological deficits are associated with lesions to the frontal lobes. The frontal lobes mediate many of the attentional processes needed for cognitive tasks (hence the inability to spell WORLD backwards or perform serial 7s) and control our ability to shift between tasks (hence perseveration emerging with frontal lobe lesions).

Hodges JR, *Cognitive Assessment for Clinicians*, Second Edition, Oxford University Press, 2007.

33. A. Dominant hemisphere

These are features of the dominant hemisphere (usually the left-hand hemisphere). These are the functions that are assessed when someone has had a stroke. Lesions to the dominant hemisphere usually render patients quite disabled as they are unable to understand instructions for rehabilitation.

Hodges JR, *Cognitive Assessment for Clinicians*, Second Edition, Oxford University Press, 2007.

34. C. Anti-Cw5

Hyperacute rejection is formed because of pre-formed antibodies to the renal graft, and anti-Cw5 antibodies have been identified as a major culprit. Antibody-antigen complexes lead to massive complement activation, capillary thrombosis, and very rapid graft loss. HLA class C matching has of course reduced the incidence of hyperacute rejection. Anti-CD3 antibodies (T-cell modulators), and anti-CD20 antibodies (B-cell-depleting agents) are used in transplant induction to reduce the risk of rejection.

Frohn C et al., The effect of HLA-C matching on acute renal transplant rejection, *Nephrology Dialysis Transplantation* 2001;16:355–360.

35. B. Aspirin overdose

The blood gas results are consistent with metabolic acidosis. In order to ascertain the cause of this type of metabolic abnormality, it is helpful to find out the degree of the anion gap. This would help stratify the types of metabolic acidosis and allows accurate management plans accordingly. One way to calculate the anion gap is to add the number of chloride and bicarbonate anions and subtract them from the number of sodium and potassium cations. $(Na^+ + K^+) - (Cl^- + HCO_3^-) =$ anion gap. The normal level of anion gap is generally considered to be between 8 and 16 mmol/L. An anion gap exceeding 24 mmol/L will suggest causes responsible for high anion gap metabolic acidosis.

Table 1.2 Metabolic acidosis

High anion gap metabolic acidosis	Normal anion gap metabolic acidosis
Lactic acidosis	GI alkali loss (diarrhoea, ileostomy, colostomy)
Ketoacidosis	Renal tubular acidosis (types 1, 2, and 4)
Intoxication (ethylene glycol, methanol, paraldehyde, salicylates	Interstitial renal disease
Renal failure	Acetozolamide therapy
	Ureterosigmoidostomy
	Ingestion of ammonium chloride

Gabow PA et al., Acid-base disturbances in the salicylate-intoxicated adult, *Archives of Internal Medicine* 1978;138:1481–1484.

36. A. Intravenous calcium gluconate

All of these therapies are recognized treatments for hyperkalaemia. This man, however, has life-threatening renal failure, with hyperkalaemia and ECG changes. As such calcium gluconate must be administered as soon as possible under ECG monitoring. It is usually followed with IV insulin and dextrose and potentially nebulized salbutamol whilst the cause of the renal failure is elucidated.

Longmore M et al., *Oxford Handbook of Clinical Medicine*, Eighth Edition, Oxford University Press, 2010.

37. E. Hypertriglyceridaemia

Severe hypertriglyceridemia (triglyceride levels greater than [5.65 mmol/L]) may manifest as a grossly lipemic serum sample when levels exceed (10 mmol/L). Severe hypertriglyceridaemia represents an extreme of the classic blood lipid pattern in diabetes. Lipaemic samples should always prompt measurement of fasting triglyceride by the laboratory. The risk of developing pancreatitis is 1–4% over a triglyceride level of 10 mmol/L and needs urgent therapy. Statins and fibrates take many days to have full therapeutic effect. Insulin activates hormone sensitive lipase, and therefore reduces triglyceride levels by hydrolysing it to lipoproteins which are subsequently stored in the adipose tissue or oxidized. Insulin is a therapeutic option for the emergency treatment of extreme hypertriglyceridaemia. Secondary hypertriglyceridaemias include hypothyroidism, kidney abnormalities (e.g. nephrotic syndrome or chronic kidney failure), diabetes mellitus, heavy alcohol consumption, and obesity. All other disorders in the list are not associated with lipemic serum.

Brunzell JD, Bierman EL, Chylomicronemia syndrome: interaction of genetic and acquired hypertriglyceridemia, *Medical Clinics of North America* 1982;66:455–468.

38. A. Accumulation of 6-mercaptopurine due to reduced hepatic metabolism

TMPT is thiopurine s-methyl transferase, an enzyme responsible for the metabolism of thiopurines. Low TMPT activity leads to accumulation of 6-mercaptopurine, the active metabolite of azathioprine. In turn this may lead to bone marrow suppression and azathioprine toxicity. TMPT activity does not affect absorption or excretion of azathioprine or its metabolites.

Chapman S et al., *Oxford Handbook of Respiratory Medicine*, Second Edition, Oxford University Press, 2009 Chapter 54, Immunosuppressive drugs.

39. B. C4

The absence of urticaria against a background of angioedema raises the possibility of C1 inhibitor deficiency. Out of the options given, C4 is always reduced during an acute attack. First presentation normally occurs around the onset of puberty. C3 levels are normal in patients with congenital C1 inhibitor deficiency, although in acquired disease, which is related to active SLE, C3 levels may be reduced. C5–C9 form the membrane attack complex, and levels are not affected by C1 inhibitor deficiency.

Provan D, *Oxford Handbook of Clinical and Laboratory Investigation*, Third Edition, Oxford University Press, 2010, Chapter 4, Immunology & allergy.

40. B. Parmesan cheese

Brown rice, sugar, and pasta are primary sources of carbohydrate, which contains 4 calories of energy per gramme. This is similar to the energy content of protein, and thus the chicken breast. In contrast two-thirds to three-quartersof cheese is comprised of fat, which contains 9 calories of energy per gramme. As such out of the options given, parmesan cheese is the most calorie dense.

Understanding calories. http://www.nhs.uk/Livewell/loseweight/Pages/understanding-calories.aspx.

41. E. Sample haemolysis

Isolated hyperkalaemia is frequently seen where GP blood samples have been left to stand for some time, usually when they are collected from a rural location and take some time to reach the analyser. In the presence of other normal lab values, and limited clinical history only mentioning tiredness, the chances of a more significant problem are slim. In this situation it's most appropriate to ask the patient to attend the emergency department so that his potassium can be re-tested.

Warrell DA, *Oxford Textbook of Medicine*, Fifth Edition, Oxford University Press, 2010, Chapter 21, Disorders of potassium homeostasis: hyperkalaemia.

42. B. Mass spectrometry

This is a potentially common situation in drug development, where the metabolites formed as a result of use of a particular agent are not known. Whilst NMR is effective at characterizing metabolites, it measures approximately 200 known metabolites. As such, mass spectrometry is the better option, as a number of peaks, corresponding to different metabolites, can be characterized. Radioimmunoassay, or ELISA relies on knowing/suspecting what the metabolite actually is before doing the test.

Current Drug Metabolism. http://www.eurekaselect.com/56310/article.

43. C. Maternal inheritance

Mitchondrial disorders are inherited via the maternal line, because chromosomal DNA is 100% contained within the oocyte. They are responsible for a range of diseases and age of onset is variable. Examples of disorders related to mitochondrial inheritance include: blindness; developmental delay; gastrointestinal problems; hearing loss; heart rhythm problems; metabolic disturbances; and short stature. Kearns–Sayre syndrome is an example of a mitchondrial disorder which results in chronic, progressive, external ophthalmoplegia, retinopathy, and cardiac conduction abnormalities.

Elliott P et al., *Oxford Specialist Handbook of Inherited Cardiac Disorders*, Oxford University Press, 2011. Chapter 17, Mitochondrial disease.

44. B. Binds to the LDL receptor

PCSK9 (Proprotein convertase subtilisin/kexin type 9) binds to the LDL receptor leading to destruction of both the LDL receptor and the LDL cholesterol bound to it. If PCSK9 is inhibited, then the LDL receptor can return to the cell surface and bind more cholesterol. As such it is an important potential target for LDL cholesterol reduction. Monoclonal antibodies are currently in phase 3 clinical trials which bind PCSK9, leading to very large falls in LDL cholesterol on top of statin therapy. RNA anti-sense technologies are in earlier stage clinical trials, which reduce levels of PCSK9.

Steinberg D, Witztum JL, Inhibition of PCSK9: a powerful weapon for achieving ideal LDL cholesterol levels, *Proceedings of the National Academy of Sciences of the United States of America* 2009;106:9546–9547. http://www.ncbi.nlm.nih.gov/pmc/articles/PMC2701045.

45. D. It shows no difference in the target populations when there is a significant difference

When organizing a study, it is very important to ensure that the sample size is appropriate to minimize type I and type II errors. **Type I error**: There is a false conclusion that there is a significant difference between the groups under study when in fact there is not. **Type II error**: There is a false conclusion that there is no significant difference between the groups under study when in fact there is a difference.

Peacock J, Peacock P, *Oxford Handbook of Medical Statistics*, Oxford University Press, 2010, Chapter 1, Research design, p. 62.

46. B. 75% of patients weigh less than this patient

Centiles (or percentiles) divide the data into set percentages. Any percentiles can be calculated, although the lower (25th), Mid (50th) and upper (75th) are the most common.

Peacock J, Peacock P, *Oxford Handbook of Medical Statistics*, Oxford University Press, 2010, Chapter 6, Summarizing data.

47. A. 99% of subjects are within three standard deviations of the mean

When assuming *normal distribution*, 99% of subjects are within three standard deviations of the mean, 95% of subjects within two standard deviations and 68% of subjects are within one standard deviation of the mean. Z scores (not M scores) can be used instead of standard deviation to estimate distribution. If an observation lies one standard deviation away from the mean, its Z score is 1. Standard deviation is the square of *variance*.

Peacock J, Peacock P, *Oxford Handbook of Medical Statistics*, Oxford University Press, 2010, Chapter 6, Summarizing data.

48. E. Double blind crossover

To test a novel treatment a randomised control trial should be used to verify its effectiveness. A cross over study provides better results when comparing treatments but can only be used if a treatment is not disease modifying. In this case the drug is likely to be helpful in epileptics.

Peacock J, Peacock P, *Oxford Handbook of Medical Statistics*, Oxford University Press, 2010.

49. A. Paired T-Test

The best test needs to compare the average blood pressure result before and after the endoscopic procedure. A paired sample T-test will compare the means of two variables and tests to see if the average difference is significantly different from zero.

Peacock J, Peacock P, *Oxford Handbook of Medical Statistics*, Oxford University Press, 2010, Chapter 1, Research Design.

50. A. Spread of data around the median value

The Standard deviation indicates how dispersed the data are and is a measure of the average difference between the mean and each data value.

Peacock J, Peacock P, *Oxford Handbook of Medical Statistics*, Oxford University Press, 2010, Chapter 8, Statistical tests.

51. E. Meta-analysis

A Meta-analysis is a statistical analysis of a collection of studies often collected through a systemic review. As such it gives information based on many other studies. Case studies are based on individual cases. A cohort study is an observational study that aims to investigate causes of disease or factors related to a condition but, unlike a case-controlled study, it is longitudinal and starts with an unselected group of individuals who are followed up for a set period of time.

Peacock J, Peacock P, *Oxford Handbook of Medical Statistics*, Oxford University Press, 2010, Chapter 13, Metaanalysis.

Ward H et al., *Oxford Handbook of of Epidemiology for Clinicians*, Oxford University Press, 2012.

52. A. Chi-Square test

The Chi-squared tests for an association between two categorical variables where each variable has only two categories. The data can thus fit into a 2x2 table, which can be used to test whether there is an association between success and the use of sclerotherapy.

Peacock J, Peacock P, *Oxford Handbook of Medical Statistics*, Oxford University Press, 2010, Chapter 8, Statistical tests.

53. D. Nominal data

Nominal data is a categorical data type in which the groups cannot be ordered. Ordinal and nominal data are categorical data. Nominal cannot be ordered but ordinal can (e.g. very happy, happy, unhappy). Continuous and discrete data are numerical.

Peacock J, Peacock P, *Oxford Handbook of Medical Statistics*, Oxford University Press, 2010, Chapter 8, Statistical tests.

54. A. 25–75%

The interquartile range of values include the middle 50% of values and is bounded by the lower (25%) and upper (75%) quartile.

Peacock J, Peacock P, *Oxford Handbook of Medical Statistics*, Oxford University Press, 2010, Chapter 6, Summarizing data, p. 183.

55. A. It increases with increasing enzyme concentration

The single defining property of the V_{max} value is that it increases with increasing enzyme concentration. The higher the enzyme concentration, the more active sites there are at which the reaction can occur (provided there is adequate substrate). This is the basis of an assay of enzyme activity. A competitive inhibitor (B) has no effect on V_{max}, whereas a non-competitive inhibitor (D) reduces it. The K_m is a measure of the affinity of enzyme active sites for the substrate and has units of concentration (mmol/L). The concentration at which V_{max} occurs is not twice the K_m (C), but rather, K_m is the substrate concentration at $\frac{1}{2} V_{max}$. The units of V_{max} are those of a rate, not a concentration (E).

Peacock J, Peacock P, *Oxford Handbook of Medical Statistics*, Oxford University Press, 2010, Chapter 1, Research Design.

56. D. It forms a covalent complex with the enzyme

The other statements typify competitive inhibitors, which form the other class of inhibitors of enzyme-catalysed reactions. By reacting with the enzyme for an extended or indefinite period of time, a non-competitive inhibitor irreversibly reduces the activity of the enzyme. Penicillin is a good example, inhibiting a critical enzyme (transpeptidase) required for bacterial cell wall synthesis; the action of aspirin on the enzyme cyclo-oxygenase to reduce infl ammation is another.

Peacock J, Peacock P, *Oxford Handbook of Medical Statistics*, Oxford University Press, 2010, Chapter 1, Research Design.

57. C. Ganglioside

Complex oligosaccharides are covalently linked to the sphingolipid component of gangliosides. Cerebrosides (A) are also glycosphingolipids, but they have only a simple sugar (glucose or galactose). Phosphatidylinositol (D) contains the simple carbohydrate inositol. Sphingomyelin (E) is a membrane lipid that contains no carbohydrate; nor does cholesterol (B). Cholera toxins bind to gangliosides in the cell membrane of the intestinal epithelium. Toxins then enter the cell, causing the secretion of anions (notably chloride) into the intestinal lumen. Water then follows the anions into the intestinal lumen by osmosis leading to the profound secretory diarrhoea that characterizes cholera infection.

Peacock J, Peacock P, *Oxford Handbook of Medical Statistics*, Oxford University Press, 2010, Chapter 1, Research Design.

58. C. Opening of ion channels

Binding of the ligand, acetylcholine, to the nicotinic receptor at the neuromuscular junction (NMJ) opens a channel that allows the passage of cations (sodium and potassium ions) across the plasma membrane. Potassium leaves the cell and sodium enters, both moving along their respective concentration gradients. The result is depolarization of the membrane of the skeletal muscle fibre, producing an end-plate potential, as the membrane voltage moves to a value halfway between the sodium and potassium equilibrium potentials. This depolarization leads in turn to Ca_2+ release (D) from the sarcoplasmic reticulum followed by muscle fibre contraction. The opening of the ion channels is extremely rapid, faster than could be achieved by an enzyme-dependent process (e.g. protein kinase as in A), by protein synthesis involving gene transcription (B) or by synthesis of a second messenger (E).

Peacock J, Peacock P, *Oxford Handbook of Medical Statistics*, Oxford University Press, 2010, pp. 50–51, Figure 1.30.

59. B. Dysplasia

Dysplasia is abnormal tissue growth and represents a premalignant condition. Note that the epithelial cells are becoming disorganized with more deeply staining (hyperchromatic) and irregularly shaped (pleomorphic) nuclei. At this stage the cells have not yet breached the basement membrane. Anaplasia (A) is a loss of cellular differentiation; hyperplasia (C) is an abnormal increase in cell number; metaplasia (D) is transformation of one tissue type into the appearance of another; neoplasia (E) is formation of new cells that may produce a cancer.

Peacock J, Peacock P, *Oxford Handbook of Medical Statistics*, Oxford University Press, 2010, pp. 75.

60. E. Tumour suppressor gene loss

Retinoblastoma is a rare childhood tumour of the eye. Most cases present within the first three years of life and are sporadic. The condition may affect one or both eyes. About 20% of unilateral cases and all bilateral tumours are believed to be hereditary. The hereditary form of retinoblastoma tends to present earlier than the sporadic disease. Retinoblastoma is caused by a mutation in a tumour suppressor gene that prevents its normal expression. Such 'loss of function' mutations contribute to the development of cancer by inactivating the normal inhibition of cell growth provided by tumour suppressor gene proteins. Oncogenes encode proteins that control cell proliferation, apoptosis, or both. Activation or amplification of oncogenes by mutations, gene amplification, or chromosomal rearrangements can therefore lead to increased cell proliferation or increased cell survival of cells carrying such alterations. The activation leads to either a structural alteration in the oncogene or an increase in, or deregulation of, its expression. Many cancers are caused by alterations in oncogenes. For example, activating point mutations occur in a substantial proportion of melanomas. Amplification of MYC has been found in small cell lung cancer, breast cancer, oesophageal cancer, and many others. Chromosomal rearrangements leading to oncogenic activity are common in prostate cancer.

Croce C, Oncogenes and cancer, *New England Journal of Medicine* 2008;3:502–511.

61. C. Gain of one homologous chromosome

Rocker-bottom foot is highly suggestive of Edwards' syndrome. This syndrome results from the presence of the usual two copies of chromosome 18 plus an additional copy, a condition known as trisomy 18. Chromosomal abnormalities can be broadly divided into numerical (e.g. aneuploidy—such as trisomy 21, known as Down's syndrome—or polyploidy) and structural (translocations, deletions, as in option D, or insertions). Single-gene abnormalities due to a mutation in a gene which codes for a specific protein may arise due to deletion of bases (B) as in Duchenne muscular dystrophy. A mutation in a gene may also cause insertion of bases (as in haemophilia A), or substitution of one base for a different base (E) as occurs in sickle-cell anaemia. Trinucleotide repeat diseases, such as Fragile X syndrome or Huntington's disease (chorea), are characterized by amplification (that is repeated copies) of a specific trinucleotide sequence (A) in a gene.

Peacock J, Peacock P, *Oxford Handbook of Medical Statistics*, Oxford University Press, 2010, Chapter 7, Probability and distributions.

62. C. Mitochondrial

A woman's ovum contributes all the mitochondria of the zygote at fertilization; the man's sperm makes no such contribution. Hence any gene on the mitochondrial DNA is inherited from the mother (maternal inheritance), and all the children of an affected woman will themselves inherit the condition. For genes on the nuclear DNA, no such pattern of inheritance is expected. A man with an autosomal dominant (A) condition will (on average) pass on the mutant gene, and hence the disease, to half his children. A woman with an autosomal recessive (B) disease will most likely have all heterozygous children who are clinically normal. Most X-linked (D) genetic disorders are inherited in a recessive manner, with a female carrier passing on the mutant gene, and hence the disease, to half her sons. The rare Y-linked (E) genetic conditions are only transmitted from father to son.

Peacock J, Peacock P, *Oxford Handbook of Medical Statistics*, Oxford University Press, 2010, pp. 158, 206.

63. E. Ventral root

The patient presents with no sensory disability but only motor symptoms. This indicates that the sensory input is intact and therefore rules out the dorsal root (A), peripheral nerves (C), and spinal nerves (D) as possible sites of injury. Since an electromyogram (EMG) can be recorded, both nerve conduction and muscle contraction are present and the neuromuscular junctions (B) are functioning, although the compound muscle action potential (CMAP) is reduced in size. The most likely explanation is a problem in a ventral root on the right side of the body causing selective loss of motor axons which results in a smaller EMG. Loss of some motor axons does not affect the conduction velocity of the nerve, just the size of CMAP.

Peacock J, Peacock P, *Oxford Handbook of Medical Statistics*, Oxford University Press, 2010, pp. 216, 252.

64. B. Grey ramus

Sympathetic autonomic neurones have cell bodies in the lateral horn of the spinal cord grey matter and their myelinated axons pass out of the cord via the ventral root (D) of the spinal nerve and through the white ramus (E) to the paravertebral ganglia. Many preganglionic fibres synapse here with postsynaptic unmyelinated fibres, while other preganglionic sympathetic fibres pass directly through the paravertebral ganglia and synapse in the prevertebral ganglian (the superior mesenteric, inferior mesenteric, and coeliac ganglia) or the adrenal medulla. The sympathetic chain (C) contains a mixture of preganglionic and postganglionic axons. The dorsal root (A) is sensory and contains both myelinated and unmyelinated fibres entering the spinal cord. The grey ramus contains only unmyelinated postganglionic axons. These pass from the paravertebral ganglion through the white ramus before joining other myelinated and unmyelinated fibres in the spinal nerve. Sympathetic postganglionic fibres taking this route innervate blood vessels of skin and muscle, sweat glands, and the pilomotor muscles of hair.

Peacock J, Peacock P, *Oxford Handbook of Medical Statistics*, Oxford University Press, 2010, Chapter 7, Probability and distributions.

65. D. Inactivation of the voltage-dependent sodium channels

When an axon is depolarized to the threshold voltage there is a dramatic increase in the sodium permeability of the membrane, allowing sodium influx (E) along both concentration (high external sodium) and electrochemical attraction (cell inside negative) gradients. In one of the few positive feedback processes known in cells, this sodium influx causes further depolarization, leading to greater sodium permeability, and yet more sodium entry. The change in membrane voltage rapidly accelerates to a point close to the sodium equilibrium potential (E_{Na}). Before the resting membrane potential can be restored, the high sodium permeability must be switched off and the membrane potential must be moved back towards E_K. The voltage-dependent sodium channels activated at threshold show spontaneous closure once they have been depolarized for a millisecond or so. This inactivation of the sodium channels occurs at the peak of the action potential. By this time the depolarization of the membrane has also brought about opening of voltage-dependent potassium channels which now allow an efflux of positively charged potassium ions (B), again driven by electrochemical and concentration gradients. This efflux moves membrane voltage in a negative direction towards the resting membrane potential. The higher-than-normal potassium permeability causes an undershoot (hyperpolarization) of the membrane voltage (C). The negative membrane voltage now closes the voltage-dependent potassium channels and the resting potassium permeability is restored producing the resting membrane potential once again. Active sodium pumping (A) maintains the low internal sodium and high internal potassium concentrations required for the above processes, but does not contribute directly to each action potential.

Peacock J, Peacock P, *Oxford Handbook of Medical Statistics*, Oxford University Press, 2010, Chapter 7, Probability and distributions.

66. C. Middle meningeal artery

The pterion is the junction between four bones at the temple (squamous temporal, greater wing of sphenoid, parietal, and frontal) and is the weakest part of the skull. It may be fractured either by a direct blow, or through an indirect impact of sufficient force to injure this weakest point. The middle meningeal artery is closely related to the pterion and can be ruptured by a fracture here. This leads to a build-up of blood between the skull and the dura mater, which is an extradural haematoma. This can cause increased intracranial pressure leading to unconsciousness and death. Extradural haematomas are arterial and so evolve rapidly, whereas subdural haematomas, where blood gathers between the dura mater and the arachnoid mater, are normally venous and therefore evolve more slowly. The superficial temporal artery (D) ascends over the temple superficial to the skull. A cerebral aneurysm of the middle cerebral artery (B) would lead to a subarachnoid haemorrhage. The cavernous sinus (A) and transverse sinus (E) are parts of a system of venous sinuses that drain blood from the internal and external veins of the brain and also collect cerebrospinal fluid. Head trauma can lead to dural venous thrombosis—a rare type of stroke.

Peacock J, Peacock P, *Oxford Handbook of Medical Statistics*, Oxford University Press, 2010.

67. D. Subarachnoid haemorrhage

The subarachnoid space surrounds the brain and the spinal cord, between the arachnoid membrane and the pia mater. It is the cavity in which cerebrospinal fluid (CSF) is contained and is the interface between the vasculature and the CSF. A subarachnoid haemorrhage (SAH), which is a form of stroke, is bleeding into this space. SAH may occur as a result of a head injury, but more commonly occurs due to a ruptured cerebral aneurysm, particularly around the circle of Willis. SAH symptoms include a severe headache, which can have a very rapid onset ('a thunderclap headache'). Other symptoms can include vomiting, an altered state of consciousness, and, sometimes, seizures. A head CT scan will correctly diagnose an SAH in the majority of cases and so should be performed immediately. If the CT is negative and an SAH is suspected, a lumbar puncture is performed. The arachnoid layer and subarachnoid space are continuous throughout the spinal cord, and so CSF sampled from the lumbar puncture can show evidence of haemorrhage. Cerebral venous sinus thrombosis (A) is a clot within the dural sinuses. In CT scans, an extradural haematoma (B) is normally seen as a convex-lens-shaped depression between the skull and the dura mater. The subdural space is not continuous around the spinal cord. An intracerebral haemorrhage (C) occurs when blood leaks directly into the brain. Subdural haematomas (E) collect between the outer meningeal layers (the dura and the arachnoid mater).

Ward H et al., *Oxford Handbook of of Epidemiology for Clinicians*, Oxford University Press, 2012, pp. 482–483.

68. C. 8

The GCS is used to assess consciousness in adults. It includes three parameters: motor function (6 grades), verbal response (5 grades) and eye opening (4 grades). A total score is the sum of the individual scores from each parameter. A score of 8 or less indicates severe injury, a score of 9–12 is associated with moderate injury, and a score of 13–15 implies minor injury. The lowest possible score is 3, while the highest is 15. In the case scenario, the GCS would be as follows: the best motor response—'Withdraws to pain' scores 4; the best verbal response—'Incomprehensible speech' scores 2; and eye opening—'Eye opening in response to pain' scores 2. Therefore, the overall score is 8, which indicates severe injury.

Teasdale G, Jennett B, Assessment of coma and impaired consciousness: a practical scale, *Lancet* 1974;304(7872):81–84.

69. C. Procedural

Memory is divided into declarative (explicit) and non-declarative (implicit) memory. Procedural memory, a type of non-declarative memory, is implicated in the acquisition of skills and habits. In Huntington's disease, damage to the striatum impairs the procedural memory of motor task learning (e.g. the ability to ride a bike without working out how to do it) without affecting declarative memory. Declarative memory (A) refers to the formation and retrieval of explicit past memories of facts and events. It is divided into episodic and semantic memory. Episodic memory (B) refers to the recollection of specific events occurring at a particular time and place (e.g. recollection of the bike route). Semantic memory (D) refers to the memory of meanings, understanding, and general knowledge unrelated to specific experiences (e.g. knowledge that a bike is for riding). Working memory (E) is a form of memory used for the short-term retention of information important for problem solving or reasoning (e.g. that the padlock key is in the garage).

Peacock J, Peacock P, *Oxford Handbook of Medical Statistics*, Oxford University Press, 2010.

1. **A 56-year-old woman with terminal breast cancer and spinal
    metastases comes to the emergency department. She complains
    of lower back pain and neuopathic pain going down her left leg.
    Current analgesia includes paracetamol and oramorph. On examination
    her BP is 145/82, pulse is 85 and regular, and she looks in pain. Her BMI
    is 22. She complains of pain on palpation of the lumbar spine and on
    raising the left leg. There are absent ankle jerks and numbness over the
    left great toe. Which of the following is the most appropriate next step
    with respect to analgesia?**
    A. Increased oramorph
    B. Amitriptilline
    C. Diclofenac
    D. Diazepam
    E. IV inbandronate

2. **A 64-year-old man presents to the clinic with night sweats, anorexia,
    and weight loss accompanied by widespread lymphadenopathy including
    the cervical region, both axillae and groins. On examination his BP is
    122/72, his pulse is 72 and regular, and his BMI is 20. You confirm the
    lymph node enlargement. Investigations: Hb 10.9, WCC 9.8, PLT 142,
    Na 138, K 4.3, Cr 121, ALT 102, ESR 95. Which of the following is
    the most appropriate investigation?**
    A. Biopsy of groin lymph node
    B. Aspiration of cervical lymph node
    C. Biopsy of cervical lymph node
    D. Bone marrow biopsy
    E. Bone marrow aspiration

3. **A 30-year-old man with haemophilia attends your office enquiring about the chances of his male offspring getting the same disease. You answer would be:**

   A. 0%

   B. 25%

   C. 50%

   D. 100%

   E. Difficult to predict

4. **A 50-year-old woman was referred with prolonged PT (INR) and normal PTT. The most likely abnormality in the coagulation screen is?**

   A. Defective factor VIII

   B. Decreased factor IX

   C. Factor VII deficiency

   D. Decreased factor XI

   E. Lupus anticoagulant

5. **A woman who is 36 weeks pregnant with her second child comes to the clinic complaining that despite only a minor knock to her left shin on a child's toy, she has sustained quite a severe bruise. Her pregnancy has been normal so far, and clinical examination reveals a BP of 121/68, her abdomen is consistent with a 36-week pregnancy. Bloods are normal apart from a platelet count which is low at 65. Which of the following is the correct intervention?**

   A. High-dose prednisolone

   B. Low-dose prednisolone

   C. No intervention is necessary

   D. Platelet transfusion

   E. Immunoglobulin transfusion

6. **A 44-year-old premenopausal woman is referred to her local gastroenterology outpatient clinic. During routine investigations, her GP has noted haemoglobin of 11.4 (normal female 12.0–16.0 g/dl), MCV 78 (normal 78–102 fl), and ferritin 9 (18–200 mcg/l). Her GP has already checked coeliac serology (negative result). She has no other major symptoms and feels otherwise well. Her mother was diagnosed with colorectal carcinoma aged 60 and required a right hemicolectomy. There is no other family history of carcinoma. What is the next most appropriate management strategy? Select the single most appropriate response.**

    A. Iron replacement
    B. Barium enema
    C. Colonoscopy
    D. Gastroscopy and colonoscopy
    E. No investigation or treatment required

7. **A 22-year-old man has been troubled by fatigue for six months. Blood tests performed by his GP reveal haemoglobin of 11.5 (normal male 13.5–18.0 g/dl), MCV 75 (normal 76–96 fl), and ferritin 11 (male 30–233 mcg/l). He has no other major symptoms and feels otherwise well. He denies relevant family history. What is the next most appropriate management strategy? Select the single most appropriate response.**

    A. Iron replacement
    B. Gastroscopy
    C. Colonoscopy
    D. Check coeliac serology
    E. No investigation or treatment required

8. **A 52-year-old postmenopausal woman is referred to her local gastroenterology outpatient clinic. During routine investigations, her GP has detected that her haemoglobin is within the normal range, but her serum ferritin is low at 12 (female 18–200 mcg/l). Her GP has already checked coeliac serology (negative result). What is the next most appropriate investigative strategy? Select the single most appropriate response.**

   A. Urgent gastroscopy
   B. None required
   C. Colonoscopy and gastroscopy
   D. Barium enema
   E. CT colonography

9. **A 21-year-old woman has undergone a splenectomy after a motorcycling accident. She has a past history of asthma and was given a pneumococcal vaccination some two years earlier. Which of the following is the current UK advice with respect to prophylaxis against pneumococcus?**

   A. Penicillin V 500 mg BD
   B. Penicillin V 250 mg BD
   C. Penicillin is not indicated
   D. Pneumococcal vaccination should be repeated every ten years
   E. She should be re-vaccinated immediately against pneumococcus

10. **A 52-year-old postmenopausal woman is referred to her local gastroenterology outpatient clinic. During routine investigations, her GP has detected that her haemoglobin is within the normal range, but her serum ferritin is low at 12 (female 18–200 mcg/l). What is the next most appropriate investigation? Select the single most appropriate response.**

    A. Urgent gastroscopy
    B. Check coeliac serology
    C. Colonoscopy
    D. Barium enema
    E. CT colonography

11. **You are looking after a patient with newly diagnosed Hodgkin's lymphoma, and he asks you about his prognosis. You are still awaiting the histology. Which of the following types on histology has the poorest prognosis?**
    A. Nodular sclerosing
    B. Mixed cellularity
    C. Lymphocyte-rich
    D. Lymphocyte-depleted
    E. All the same prognosis

12. **You request a blood film on a patient with macrocytosis. It shows megaloblastic cells. Of the choices below, which is the most likely cause of the abnormality?**
    A. Alcohol
    B. Hypothyroidism
    C. Pregnancy
    D. Liver disease
    E. Vitamin B12 deficiency

13. **A 29-year-old woman comes to the clinic two months after a second pulmonary embolus and announces that she has missed her period and has a positive pregnancy test. You wonder what to do with respect to her warfarin therapy. Which of the following is the correct advice?**
    A. Switch to LMW heparin until week 12
    B. Switch to LMW heparin after week 12
    C. Switch to LMW heparin immediately
    D. Switch to LMW heparin after week 24
    E. Switch to LMW heparin until week 24

14. **A 34-year-old woman is receiving a four-unit blood transfusion for a post-partum haemorrhage after the birth of her third child. A short time after beginning the transfusion she becomes acutely short of breath with saturations of 89% on air. Her temperature is 38 °C, BP is 100/50, pulse 92. There is marked wheeze on auscultation of the chest. Her Hb is 8.2, white count and platelets are normal, as are her U&Es. Chest X-ray shows bilateral pulmonary infiltrates. Which of the following is the most likely diagnosis?**

    A. Transfusion-associated lung injury (TRALI)
    B. Acute non-haemolytic transfusion reaction
    C. Cardiogenic pulmonary oedema.
    D. Acute haemolytic reaction
    E. IgD-mediated transfusion reaction

15. **A 58-year-old woman presents with back pain, thirst, and constipation. She is taking no drugs. Investigations reveal: Urea 19.8 mmol/l, serum potassium 5.2 mmol/l, serum creatinine 231 micromol/l, TSH 2.01 mIU/l, haemoglobin 9.9 g/dl. Ultrasound of her abdomen was normal. Which of the following is the most likely cause of her renal failure?**

    A. Acute glomerulonephritis
    B. Acute tubular necrosis
    C. Interstitial nephritis
    D. Myeloma
    E. Retroperitoneal fibrosis

16. **A 32-year-old woman becomes extremely unwell a few minutes after beginning a blood transfusion. She is hypotensive with a BP of 85/60, a pulse of 95, and looks extremely flushed. Auscultation of the chest reveals significant wheeze. Apparently there are two patients on the ward with similar names. Which of the following is the most likely diagnosis?**

    A. Febrile non-haemolytic transfusion reaction
    B. Rhesus incompatibility
    C. Bacterial infection of the unit
    D. Transfusion-related lung injury
    E. Volume overload

17. **A 70-year-old man is coming to the end of the second unit of a two-unit blood transfusion when he becomes pyrexial 38.5°C. His BP is maintained at 141/83 and his pulse is stable at 85. You give him some paracetamol and his fever settles over the next few hours. Investigations: Haemoglobin 9.7 g/dl (13.5–17.7), white cells 9.1 x 10⁹/l (4–11), platelets 234 x 10⁹/l (150–400), sodium 144 mmol/l (135–146), potassium 4.7 mmol/l (3.5–5), creatinine 141 micromol/l (79–118). Which of the following is the most likely diagnosis?**

    A. Febrile non-haemolytic transfusion reaction
    B. Rhesus incompatibility
    C. Graft versus host transfusion reaction
    D. ABO incompatibility
    E. Bacterial contamination of the unit

18. **A 56-year-old man presents with sudden onset, severe headache. He has a past history of hypertension and atrial fibrillation, for which he takes warfarin. Of note he has a family history of 'kidney trouble' and reports that several of his relatives require regular dialysis. He is admitted from accident and emergency to the medical admissions ward for further investigations. On review later that evening he is found to be drowsy with a Glasgow Coma Score of 12/15. Urgent computed tomography scan of the head reveals evidence of subarachnoid bleeding. His international normalized ratio (INR) is 2.1. Which of the following is the most appropriate initial intervention?**

    A. 10 mg intravenous vitamin K
    B. 10 mg oral vitamin K
    C. Prothrombin complex concentrate
    D. Fresh frozen plasma
    E. Tranexamic acid

19. **A 52-year-old postmenopausal woman is referred to her local gastroenterology outpatient clinic. During routine investigations, her GP has detected that her haemoglobin is within the normal range, but her serum ferritin is low at 12 (female 18–200 mcg/l). Her GP has already checked coeliac serology (negative result). Colonoscopy and gastroscopy are undertaken: both are reported to be normal. What is the next most appropriate management strategy? Select the single most appropriate response.**

    A. Iron replacement
    B. Small bowel imaging (such as small bowel barium follow through)
    C. Video capsule endoscopy
    D. Enteroscopy
    E. No investigation or treatment required

20. **A 44-year-old premenopausal woman is referred to her local gastroenterology outpatient clinic. During routine investigations, her GP has noted haemoglobin of 11.7 (normal female 12.0–16.0 g/dl), MCV 76 (normal 78–102 fl) and ferritin 6 (18–200 mcg/l). She has no other major symptoms and feels otherwise well. She denies relevant family history. What is the next most appropriate management strategy? Select the single most appropriate response.**

    A. Iron replacement
    B. Small bowel imaging (such as small bowel barium follow through)
    C. Gastroscopy and colonoscopy
    D. No investigation or treatment required
    E. Check coeliac serology

21. **A 72-year-old woman is attending for regular blood transfusions. She is currently being treated with fludarabine for chronic lymphocytic leukaemia, but is having problems with persistent anaemia, her most recent Hb being only 6.9 g/dl. She is thought to have both autoimmune haemolytic anaemia and bone marrow failure. What is the optimal way to replace her red cells?**

    A. Whole blood
    B. Whole blood through a white cell filter
    C. Whole blood with prednisolone and anti-histamine cover
    D. Red cells only
    E. Irradiated red cells

22. **A 28-year-old woman is admitted with her third attack in the past four years of severe abdominal pain, vomiting, and hyponatraemia. In addition, she is confused and agitated. The surgeons ask you to see her as whilst she was admitted with possible acute abdomen, that does not appear to be the case now. On examination her BP is 155/80, and whilst her abdomen is soft, she is suffering from diffuse pain. Bloods reveal a sodium of 129 mmol/l. Urinary coporphobilinogen is elevated, stool porphyrins are within the normal range. Which of the following is the most likely diagnosis?**
    A. Acute intermittent porphyria
    B. Variegate porphyria
    C. Hereditary coproporphyria
    D. Porphyria cutanea tarda
    E. Erythropoietic protoporphyria

23. **A 62-year-old woman presents with large volume haematemesis. She has a background of primary biliary cirrhosis and is known to have oesophageal varices. In accident and emergency (A&E) she is haemodynamically unstable with ongoing large-volume haematemesis. During her stay in A&E she receives 12 units of blood in a period of 30 minutes. Which of the following is not a recognized complication of massive red cell transfusion?**
    A. Hyperkalaemia
    B. Hypercalcaemia
    C. Metabolic acidosis
    D. Thrombocytopaenia
    E. Hypothermia

24. You are called urgently to see a 33-year-old woman who has received the third unit of a three-unit blood transfusion for post-partum haemorrhage a few hours earlier. She is short of breath and has begun to develop a chronic nagging cough which is not relieved by her salbutamol inhaler. Her O_2 saturation is reduced at 92% on air. Investigations: Haemoglobin 8.5 g/dl (11.5–16.5), white cells 8.7 x 10^9/l (4–11), platelets 197 x 10^9/l (150–400), sodium 140 mmol/l (135–146), potassium 4.7 mmol/l (3.5–5), creatinine 111 micromol/l (79–118). Which of the following is the most likely diagnosis?

    A. ABO incompatibility
    B. Rhesus incompatibility
    C. Transfusion-related lung injury
    D. Febrile non-haemolytic transfusion reaction
    E. Allergic reaction to constituents of the unit

25. A 51-year-old man who has liver impairment is undergoing a platelet transfusion. He completes the first unit without problem, but after the end of the second unit he develops rigors and a pyrexia of 38.7 °C. His BP also falls to 95/65, with an increase in his pulse to 92 BPM. His urine is negative for blood. You order some urgent blood tests which are given below: Haemoglobin 13.2 g/dl (13.5–18.5), white cells 11.9 x 10^9/l (4–11), platelets 39 x 10^9/l (150–400), sodium 138 mmol/l (135–146), potassium 4.3 mmol/l (3.5–5), creatinine 110 micromol/l (79–118). Which of the following is the most likely cause of his symptoms?

    A. Bacterial contamination of the platelet unit
    B. Viral contamination of the platelet unit
    C. White blood cells within the platelet unit
    D. ABO incompatibility
    E. Rhesus incompatibility

26. A 29-year-old woman presents with disseminated intravascular coagulopathy and is diagnosed with acute promyelocytic leukaemia. What is the most common chromosomal abnormality underlying acute promyelocytic leukaemia?

    A. t(15;17)
    B. inv(16)
    C. t(8;14)
    D. t(11;14)
    E. t(9;22)(q34;q11)

27. **A 56-year-old presents to the clinic with a rapidly enlarging lymph node on the left-hand side of her neck. She has also been suffering from increasing night sweats over the past few weeks and has lost 5 kg in weight over the past three months. On examination she looks pale; her BMI is 22. She has a lymph node enlargement on both sides of her neck and in her axillae. She has a normochromic normocytic anaemia. LDH is elevated. Which of the following is the investigation most appropriate to confirm the diagnosis?**

    A. Lymph node biopsy
    B. Fine needle aspiration biopsy
    C. Bone marrow biopsy
    D. Beta 2 microglobulin
    E. CT neck and chest

28. **A patient presents with weight loss, fever, and night sweats, and is found to have cervical lymphadenopathy. He has a lymph node biopsy showing cells consistent with Hodgkin's lymphoma, and a CT showing involvement only of a single lymph node region in the left cervical area. According to the Ann Arbor system, what stage does this patient fall in to?**

    A. IB
    B. IIA
    C. IIB
    D. IIIB
    E. IVA

29. **A 33-year old woman is admitted with acute confusion and renal impairment. A blood film shows evidence of a microangiopathic haemolytic anaemia and thrombocytopaenia. What is the underlying molecular process?**

    A. Inhibition of factor VIII
    B. Inhibition of ADAMTS13
    C. Glucose-6-phosphate dehydrogenase deficiency
    D. Mutation in janus kinase 2
    E. Acquired C1 esterase inhibitor deficiency

30. **A 17 year old woman of North African ethnic origin has been diagnosed by her GP as suffering from a urinary tract infection. She is prescribed a week's course of antibiotics but her health deteriorates some 4–5 days later with lower back pain, abdominal pain, and haematuria. Investigations reveal an Hb of 9.2 g/dL with evidence of haemolysis. Which of the following antibiotics is she most likely to have been prescribed?**

    A. Amoxycillin
    B. Ciprofloxacin
    C. Cephalexin
    D. Trimethoprim
    E. Co-amoxiclav

31. **A 50-year-old man presents to the clinic with cervical and axillary lymphadenopathy. Unfortunately, excision biopsy of one of the nodes is suggestive of diffuse large B-cell lymphoma. Which of the following features would be associated with an unfavourable prognosis?**

    A. Age 50
    B. Normal LDH
    C. BCL-2 expression
    D. BCL-6 expression
    E. Normal beta-2 microglobulin

32. **A 56-year-old man is diagnosed with a gastric lymphoma, and he is started on imatinib therapy. Which of the following correctly describes the mode of action of imatinib?**

    A. Serine kinase inhibitor
    B. Tyrosine kinase inhibitor
    C. Histidine kinase inhibitor
    D. Mixed kinase inhibitor
    E. Serine kinase inhibitor

33. **A 56-year-old woman with membranous nephropathy and nephrotic syndrome comes to the emergency department complaining that her right leg is even more swollen than usual. She has 4 g/24hrs protein loss in her urine on average, and an ultrasound scan confirms a right leg DVT. Which of the following is the most likely cause?**
    A. Protein S deficiency
    B. Anti-phospholipid antibody syndrome
    C. Factor V Leiden mutation
    D. Vitamin K deficiency
    E. Polycythaemia

34. **A 20-year-old woman comes to the haematology clinic for review. She has developed a left-sided DVT after returning from a four-hour plane journey. Only medication of note is the oral contraceptive pill, which she has now stopped and is making alternative arrangements for contraception. Her BMI is 23. She is found to be heterozygous for the factor V Leiden mutation. Which of the following is the most appropriate duration of warfarin therapy?**
    A. One month
    B. Three months
    C. Six months
    D. One year
    E. Lifelong

35. **A 22-year-old woman presents to the clinic with gallstones. She has suffered increasing abdominal pain and most recently suffered an episode of acute cholecystitis. Routine blood work up by the GP has revealed macrocytic anaemia. LDH and unconjugated bilirubin are also elevated. Apparently her father suffered from a similar condition. Which of the following is the most likely diagnosis?**
    A. Hereditary spherocytosis
    B. Autoimmune haemolytic anaemia
    C. B12 deficiency
    D. Folate deficiency
    E. Myelodysplasia

36. In which of the following situations is the anti-coagulant effect of warfarin most likely to be most potentiated?

A. When used in conjunction with St John's Wort

B. When used in conjunction with carbamazepine

C. In a patient who drinks two glasses of wine each day

D. In a patient who has an acute deterioration in renal function

E. In a patient with Gilbert's syndrome

37. A 71-year-old man presents to the haematology clinic for review. He has recently moved general practitioners and has been diagnosed with a paraproteinaemia on routine blood testing. Which of the following features would not be consistent with a diagnosis of Monoclonal Gammopathy of Unknown Significance (MGUS)?

A. Serum monoclonal protein 28g/l

B. Creatinine 152

C. Bone marrow plasma cells 8%

D. Pathological fracture right femur

E. Lytic lesions on bone scan

38. A 14-year-old boy presents to the clinic for review. He has splenomegaly which is causing him significant abdominal discomfort and he wants to be considered for splenectomy. You understand that his sister underwent the operation in the previous year. Although he only has mild tiredness, his Hb is measured at 9.5g/dl, and spherocytes are seen on the blood film. The osmotic fragility test is positive. Which of the following is the most appropriate management for him?

A. Folic acid supplementation

B. Low-dose corticosteroids

C. Azathioprine

D. Splenectomy

E. Iron supplementation

39. A 62-year-old man comes to the emergency department with a severe epistaxis. Despite packing, the area continues to ooze and he is tachycardic with a BP of 105/70 and a postural drop of 20 mmHg. The treating physician elects to start him on tranexamic acid. How does tranexamic acid function?

A. Inhibits conversion of plasminogen
B. Factor X inhibitor
C. Platelet ADP receptor activator
D. Cyclo-oxygenase inhibitor
E. Vitamin K agonist

40. A 53-year-old man with a history of colonic carcinoma with an isolated hepatic metastasis presents to the emergency department with left-sided pleuritic chest pain. On examination his BP is 108/60, pulse is 93 and regular. O2 saturation is 92% on air, and auscultation of both lung fields is normal. CTPA reveals a small left-sided pulmonary embolus. Liver function testing reveals an ALT and alkaline phosphatase which are three times the upper limit of normal, and he has mild normochromic, normocytic anaemia. Which of the following is the most appropriate treatment for him?

A. Aspirin 300 mg
B. Clopidogrel 75 mg
C. Enoxiparin
D. Warfarin
E. Rivaroxaban

41. A 70-year-old woman who takes a stable dose of 2 mg/3 mg warfarin on alternate days is referred to the emergency department by her GP because her INR has been measured at 11. She tells you the duty GP prescribed some antibiotics for a urine infection which may have interfered with her warfarin. On examination there are no signs of active bleeding and her blood pressure is stable at 128/72. Which of the following is the most appropriate way to manage her warfarin therapy?

A. Do nothing and continue dosing
B. Discontinue dosing for a few days
C. Discontinue dosing for a few days and give vitamin K 1 mg IV
D. Discontinue dosing for a few days and give vitamin K 5 mg IV
E. Discontinue dosing for a few days, give vitamin K 5 mg IV and prothrombin complex concentrate

42. **A 38-year-old woman who takes the combined oral contraceptive pill is referred to the emergency department by her GP with a swollen left leg. He suspects a DVT. On examination you confirm that her left calf is 4cm larger than the right. D-dimers are elevated at 489. You are informed by the radiologist that an ultrasound cannot be done until the following morning. Which of the following is the correct course of action?**

    A. Admit for low molecular weight heparin therapy
    B. Give low molecular weight heparin and suggest she returns for an ultrasound
    C. Put on a compression stocking and suggest she returns for an ultrasound
    D. Give her 300 mg aspirin and suggest she returns for an ultrasound
    E. Tell her to rest at home and return for an ultrasound next day

43. **A 72-year-old man presents to the clinic for review. He has complained of frequent severe headaches over the past six months and most recently suffered an inferior myocardial infarction. He also complains of severe itching. Examination reveals a BP of 155/72, pulse of 75 and regular. He has a ruddy complexion and you note splenomegaly on abdominal examination. Haemoglobin is elevated at 188g/l, white count is elevated at 15.2 (4–10x10(9)/l), platelets are elevated at 672 (130–400x10(9)/l). You suspect a diagnosis of primary polycythaemia. Which of the following abnormalities is also likely to be present?**

    A. Philadelphia translocation
    B. JAK2 mutation
    C. Elevated erythropoeitin
    D. Elevated ferritin
    E. Elevated G6PD

44. **A 72-year-old man presents to the TIA clinic for review. He as a history of frequent headaches which have become worse over the past two months and he has suffered two episodes of transient left-sided facial weakness in the past three weeks. On examination his BP is 165/90, pulse is 75 and regular. He has plethoric features. Blood testing reveals an Hb of 180g/l (140–170), WCC 13.4x10(9)/l (4–10), PLT 640x10(9)/l (150–400). A diagnosis of primary polycythaemia is made and he is commenced on low-dose aspirin. Which of the following is the most appropriate initial management?**
    A. Do nothing more
    B. Add hydroxycarbamide
    C. Add phlebotomy
    D. Add clopidogrel
    E. Add dipyridamole

45. **A patient with a history of prostate cancer is admitted with symptoms suggestive of spinal cord compression. Which investigation is the most important for his rapid diagnosis and management?**
    A. Full spinal x-rays
    B. Full spinal CT scan
    C. Full spinal MRI scan
    D. PSA level
    E. Prostate biopsy

46. **A 25-year-old man presents with breathlessness, a headache worse on leaning forwards, and recurrent syncopal episodes. On examination he has a cyanotic appearance with venous distension of the face and upper body. Which investigation will best confirm the diagnosis?**
    A. Blood film.
    B. Bronchoscopy and biopsy.
    C. Chest x-ray.
    D. Contrast-enhanced computed tomography.
    E. Extrathoracic lymph node biopsy.

47. **A 45-year-old woman presents to her GP concerned about her risk of breast cancer. Her elder sister was diagnosed with carcinoma of the breast at the age of 53. She has two unaffected sisters. Her mother remains well but her maternal grandmother was diagnosed with breast cancer at the age of 67, and of her three maternal aunts, one was diagnosed with the disease at the age of 59. Which of the following statements is true, regarding the aetiology of breast cancer?**

A. Late menarche and early menopause in women are associated with an increased risk

B. Men with Klinefelter's syndrome are at three-fold increased risk

C. Evidence supports moderate daily alcohol intake as being protective against breast cancer

D. Higher socio-economic status is associated with a greater risk of breast cancer

E. Women who have inherited either *BRCA1* or *BRCA2* gene mutations have a 25% lifetime risk of developing breast cancer

48. **A 45-year-old woman presents to the clinic for review after removal of a left breast carcinoma. She is asking about long-term therapy to prevent a recurrence, and is particularly concerned because her mother was treated with tamoxifen but still suffered a further tumour, and died some three years after her original surgery. Mutations in which one of the following genes are thought to be related tamoxifen resistance?**

A. *BRCA1*

B. *BRCA2*

C. *BCAR4*

D. *BCAR3*

E. *BCAR1*

49. **A 73-year-old male presents to the acute medical take with a five-day history of nausea and constipation and 24 hours of acute confusion. On examination he is clinically dehydrated with reduced air entry in the right upper lobe and palpable hepatomegaly. His adjusted serum calcium is 3.19 mmol/l. Regarding the acute presentation of malignant hypercalcaemia:**

A. It is a common presentation of previously undiagnosed solid tumours

B. Chvostek's sign may be present

C. Treatment is usually with urgent administration of bisphosphonates, followed by steroids

D. Treatment is usually with urgent rehydration, followed by bisphosphonates

E. Treatment is usually with urgent administration of bisphosphonates, followed by rehydration and dietary calcium restriction

50. **A 21-year-old rugby player presents to accident and emergency with an acute rib injury. As part of his managment a CXR is arranged which demonstrates bilateral pulmonary opacities consistent with metastatic disease affecting the lungs. On closer questioning he admits to feeling less well for the last two months, with an irritating non-productive cough and some intermittent lower back pain. He has lost around half a stone in weight. Testicular examination confirms non-tender enlargement of the right testis. Regarding testicular cancer:**

    A. Testicular cancer accounts for only around 1% of cancers in men
    B. Acute scrotal pain is highly suggestive of malignancy
    C. 60% of cases are in patients with a history of cryptorchidism
    D. Gynaecomastia is a common finding in men with testicular cancer
    E. Symptoms of hypothyroidism may form part of the presentation of testicular cancer

51. **A 70-year-old woman comes to the clinic for evaluation of painless lymphadenopathy which has progressively increased over the past two months. Her only other past medical history of note is Type 2 diabetes for which she takes metformin 500 mg and ramipril 5 mg daily. On examination her BP is 125/72, pulse is 72 and regular. There is bilateral cervical lymphadenopathy, with several very large lymph nodes. Bloods reveal anaemia with an Hb of 10.2 g/dL, and an ESR of 78. Which of the following is the optimal investigation with respect to determining the prognosis in this patient?**

    A. Cytogenetics
    B. Bone marrow trefine
    C. Fine needle aspiration of a lymph node
    D. Excision biopsy of a lymph node
    E. PET scanning of head, neck, and thorax

CLINICAL HAEMATOLOGY AND ONCOLOGY

ANSWERS

1. B. Amitriptilline

In this situation a significant component of her pain appears to be related to nerve compression. In this situation a tricyclic antidepressant may be highly effective in improving analgesia. As such amitriptilline is the preferred answer. It is thought to work by interfering with reuptake of serotonin and noradrenaline within the dorsal horn. It may also work via sodium channel effects, NDMA inhibition, or alpha blockade. A non-steroidal may be useful in improving the bony component of the pain, if it is still not controlled with the addition of the tricyclic, as may a bisphosphonate.

Bennett M, *OPML Neuropathic Pain*, Second Edition, Oxford University Press, 2010, Chapter 9, Cancer neuropathic pain.

2. C. Biopsy of cervical lymph node

This patient's symptoms and raised ESR suggest the possibility of a lymphoid malignancy. The next investigation of choice is lymph node biopsy. Aspiration is rarely satisfactory as it does not give information about lymph node architecture. Groin lymph node changes are often non-specific and biopsy of these should therefore be avoided. Bone marrow biopsy is reserved for staging in confirmed lymphoma or leukaemia cases, and until the diagnosis of lymphoma is confirmed, and the patient has gone through CT staging, bone marrow biopsy is not appropriate. Equally bone marrow aspiration is subsidiary to lymph node investigation when there are palpable nodes.

Provan D et al., *Oxford Handbook of Clinical Haematology*, Third Edition, Oxford University Press, 2009, Chapter 1, Clinical approach, Lymphadenopathy.

3. A. 0%

Haemophilia is a serious bleeding disorder caused by a recessive mutation on the X chromosome. Because the related mutation is recessive, haemophilia is more common in boys than in girls, as boys do not have another copy of the X chromosome to compensate for the genetic defect. On the other hand, most girls born with haemophilia mutations are carriers, because they each possess only one mutated gene on one of their two X chromosomes. Although not themselves affected by haemophilia, carriers can pass haemophilia genes on to their children. An affected father passes the healthy Y chromosome to his sons while they acquire the X chromosome from their mother. Therefore unless the mother is a carrier, the sons of a haemophilic father would always escape the disease. If the father has the disease and the mother is normal, there is a 100% chance of a normal boy and a 100% chance of a carrier girl without the disease.

Provan D et al., *Oxford Handbook of Clinical Haematology*, Third Edition, Oxford University Press, 2009, Chapter 10, Haemostasis and thrombosis, Haemophilia A and B.

4. C. Factor VII deficiency

The PTT evaluates the coagulation factors XII, XI, IX, VIII, X, V, and II (prothrombin). A PT test (INR) evaluates the coagulation factors VII, X, V, II, and I (fibrinogen). Both are prolonged when the common pathway coagulation (factors X, V, II) are depleted or dysfunctional. Isolated factor VII deficiency would result in isolated prolonged PT (INR) with normal PTT. Factor VII deficiency is a rare congenital coagulation disorder transmitted with autosomal recessive inheritance. Clinical phenotypes range from asymptomatic, even in homozygotes, to severe disease characterized by life-threatening and disabling symptoms (central nervous system and gastrointestinal bleeding and haemarthrosis). In this disorder the INR is typically prolonged while the PTT is normal. Vitamin K deficiency causes deficiency of factors VII, X, IX, and prothrombin (II) as it is essential in their activation. Vitamin K deficiency usually prolongs the PT before the PTT because it first affects the activity of factor VII, whose turnover is the most rapid. Warfarin blocks the action of vitamin K, thereby reducing the vitamin K-dependent clotting factors.

Herrmann FH et al., Molecular biology and clinical manifestation of hereditary factor VII deficiency, *Seminars in Thrombosis and Hemostasis* 2000;26(4):393–400.

5. C. No intervention is necessary

Polyclonal anti-platelet antibodies are found in pregnancy, with isolated low platelets being found in around 8% of pregnancies. Rarely do platelet counts fall below 70, and epidural anaesthesia is still an option as long as platelet counts remain above 50. In this case the platelet count is well above 50, and the benefit:risk of an intervention such as corticosteroids is not justified in this case.

Provan D et al., *Oxford Handbook of Clinical Haematology*, Third Edition, Oxford University Press, 2009, Chapter 1, Clinical approach, Thrombocytopenia in pregnancy.

6. C. Colonoscopy

In this premenopausal woman with no symptoms but a relevant family history of colorectal carcinoma history, colonoscopy is the next appropriate step. Coeliac serology has already been checked, so now the priority is to rule out any large intestinal malignancy. Colonoscopy is far superior to barium enema in this situation.

British Society of Gastroenterology, Guidelines for the management of irondeficiency anaemia, 2011. http://www.bsg.org.uk/images/stories/docs/clinical/guidelines/sbn/bsg_ida_2011.pdf.

7. D. Check coeliac serology

In this young male with iron deficiency anaemia, coeliac disease should be ruled out as a first step prior to embarking upon invasive investigations.

British Society of Gastroenterology, Guidelines for the management of irondeficiency anaemia, 2011. http://www.bsg.org.uk/images/stories/docs/clinical/guidelines/sbn/iron_def.pdf.

8. C. Colonoscopy and gastroscopy

The BSG guideline is clear that, in instances of iron deficiency without anaemia, postmenopausal females should be investigated. Following negative coeliac serology, upper and lower GI investigations are recommended. This would usually be undertaken as a gastroscopy and colonoscopy, and this is clearly the most appropriate response.

British Society of Gastroenterolgy, Guidelines for the management of iron deficiency anaemia, 2005. http://www.bsg.org.uk/images/stories/docs/clinical/guidelines/sbn/iron_def.pdf.

9. A. Penicillin V 500 mg BD

The greatest risk of infection is during the two years after splenectomy, and UK guidelines recommend penicillin at least during this period. With respect to pneumococcal vaccination, it should be repeated every five years. Where there is penicillin allergy, erythromycin is the default choice.

http://www.bcshguidelines.com/documents/SPLEEN_bjh_2002.pdf.

10. B. Check coeliac serology

According to BSG guidelines, postmenopausal women and men over 50 years should be investigated if they have iron deficiency (regardless of actual anaemia or not). The first step is to rule out coeliac disease by checking coeliac serology. If this is positive, they require D2 (duodenal) biopsy on endoscopy to formally confirm the diagnosis. If coeliac is negative, then upper and lower GI endoscopy should be considered.

British Society of Gastroenterology, Guidelines for the management of iron deficiency anaemia, 2005. http://www.bsg.org.uk/images/stories/docs/clinical/guidelines/sbn/iron_def.pdf.

11. D. Lymphocyte-depleted

Hodgkin's lymphoma is a type of lymphoma characterized by the presence of Reed–Sternberg cells. These are large lymphocytes that are either multinucleated or have a bilobed nucleus, and they are sometimes said to have an 'owl's eye' appearance. It tends to initially spread via the lymphatic route and invade lymph nodes and spleen. It can also undergo haematological spread and invade other tissue such as bone marrow, liver, and lungs. The disease may be staged according to the Ann Arbor classification, with a better prognosis for patients at an earlier stage at diagnosis: (1) The lymphoma cells are in one lymph node group (or one part or tissue or organ e.g. lung); (2) The lymphoma cells are in at least two lymph node groups on the same side of the diaphragm; (3) The lymphoma cells are in lymph nodes above and below the diaphragm; (4) The lymphoma is in an organ (such as the liver, lung, or bone) and in distant lymph nodes.

Longmore M et al., *Oxford Handbook of Clinical Medicine*, Ninth Edition, Oxford University Press, 2014.

Table 2.1 Classification

Classification order of incidence *Classical Hodgkin's lymphoma*	Prognosis
Nodular sclerosing	Good
Mixed cellularity*	Good
Lymphocyte rich	Good
Lymphocyte depleted	Good

Note: nodular lymphocyte predominant Hodgkin's is recognized as a separate entity, behaving as a separate entity, behaving as an indolent B-cell lymphoma.
* Higher incidence and worse prognosis if HIV +ve
Reproduced from Longmore M. et al, *Oxford Handbook of Clinical Medicine*, Ninth Edition, 2014 with permission from Oxford University Press.

12. E. Vitamin B12 deficiency

Megaloblasts are cells in which nuclear maturation is delayed compared with the cytoplasm. In all of the above causes expect B12 deficiency, there is no delay. However, in B12 deficiency, DNA synthesis is delayed as B12 is required for this. The cells are therefore megaloblastic. Other causes of megaloblastic cells include folate deficiency and cytotoxic drugs.

Longmore M et al., *Oxford Handbook of Clinical Medicine*, Eighth Edition, Oxford University Press, 2010, Chapter 8, Haematology, Macrocytic anaemia.

13. C. Switch to LMW heparin immediately

Warfarin is unsafe after week 6 in pregnancy and during the last four weeks of pregnancy. As such switching to low molecular weight heparin is the correct answer. Occasionally, patients on long-term warfarin are switched for the final month of pregnancy, but heparin is often easier to manage, particularly if assisted delivery or caesarean section is required.

Richards D et al., *Oxford Handbook of Practical Drug Therapy*, Second Edition, Oxford University Press, 2011, Chapter 2, Cardiovascular system, Anticoagulants: Warfarin: BNF 2.8.2.

14. A. Transfusion-associated lung injury (TRALI)

This clinical picture fits best with TRALI. Two hypotheses are proposed for TRALI: that HLA antigens in the donor blood react with recipient neutrophils, or that the neutrophils do not actually need HLA antigens to react, and the process of giving birth is what primes the neutrophils to become activated. Local infiltration leads to release of cytokines and the generation of non-cardiogenic pulmonary oedema.

Provan D et al., *Oxford Handbook of Clinical Haematology*, Third Edition, Oxford University Press, 2009, Chapter 17, Blood transfusion, TRALI and TA-GVHD.

15. D. Myeloma

Thirst and abdominal pain (due to increased incidence of peptic ulceration, renal stones, pancreatitis, and constipation) in the presence of back pain are suggestive of myeloma complicated by hypercalcaemia. The thirst may be due to chronic renal disease, dehydration (secondary to tubular dysfunction following precipitation of light chains), or hypercalcaemia. Tiredness is a common symptom of myeloma secondary to anaemia +/– chronic kidney disease, and also infection. Constipation is secondary to dehydration and hypercalcaemia. Bony involvement is most common in the spine, ribs, long bones, and shoulder. X-ray appearance of myelomatous involvement of the spine may appear osteoporotic. Nuclear bone scans will not detect myelomatous involvement: a radiological skeletal survey is required.

Longmore M et al., *Oxford Handbook of Clinical Medicine*, Eighth Edition, Oxford University Press, 2010, Chapter 8, Haematology, Myeloma.

16. B. Rhesus incompatibility

The clue is that there are two patients on the ward with similar names. The rapid onset of symptoms including significant hypotension is a strong pointer towards a major problem with the transfusion either with respect to ABO or rhesus incompatibility. Febrile non-haemolytic transfusion reactions may be related to cytokines within the donor unit. Increased risk of febrile reactions occurs if people donate during a systemic illness such as a cold. Bacterial infection of the unit would lead to symptoms of hypotension, tachycardia, and fever slightly later in the transfusion process, due to exposure to bacterial lipopolysaccaride. It would certainly be a differential here in the absence of similar patient names. TRALI is thought to result from antibodies to donor HLA antigens and occurs usually in women who have received multiple blood transfusions. It leads to the development of non-cardiogenic pulmonary oedema. Given we are not given a history of multiparity, it seems unlikely here. Volume overload would not be expected to result in hypotension, and here the flushing, tachycardia, and hypotension is more likely to be related to a systemic immune response.

Massey E et al., *Practical Transfusion Medicine*, Wiley, 2009, Chapter 7, Haemolytic transfusion reactions. http://onlinelibrary.wiley.com/doi/10.1002/9781444311761.ch7/summary.

17. A. Febrile non-haemolytic transfusion reaction

Febrile non-haemolytic transfusion reactions are relatively common, and occur in around 1–2% of transfusions. Antibodies to white cells or cytokines found in the donated unit of blood are thought to be the cause. These reactions settle spontaneously with conservative management and supportive care such as anti-pyretics where required.

Heddle N, Pathophysiology of febrile nonhemolytic transfusion reactions, *Current Opinion in Hematology* 1999;6:420. http://journals.lww.com/co-hematology/Abstract/1999/11000/ Pathophysiology_of_febrile_nonhemolytic.12.aspx.

18. C. Prothrombin complex concentrate

This gentleman's history of hypertension and subarachnoid haemorrhage, in combination with a family history of renal disease, should make you think about the possibility of underlying autosomal dominant polycystic kidney disease. The patient clearly has life-threatening bleeding and requires immediate correction of his clotting. In situations with 'life or limb'-threatening bleeding (intracranial, intraocular, compartment syndrome, pericardial) this is most appropriately done with prothrombin complex concentrates such as Beriplex®. This should be performed regardless of his INR. All of the other options may be used with bleeding or coagulopathy, but given the severity of the bleeding in this case they would not be appropriate, since both vitamin K and FFP take several hours to reduce the INR and administration of vitamin K (10 mg intravenously) does not normalize the INR for 6 to 24 hours.

Aguilar MR et al., Treatment of warfarin-associated intracerebral haemorrhage: literature review and expert opinion, *Mayo Clinic Proceedings* 2007;82(1):82–92.

19. A. Iron replacement

Following normal upper and lower GI investigations, iron replacement is all that is required as long as anaemia is not transfusion dependent. If a patient has transfusion-dependent anaemia (e.g. requires transfusion every few weeks or months), then the following step would be video capsule endoscopy. This is quicker and less invasive than enteroscopy for the patient.

British Society of Gastroenterology, Guidelines for the management of iron deficiency anaemia, 2005. http://www.bsg.org.uk/images/stories/docs/clinical/guidelines/sbn/iron_def.pdf.

20. E. Check coeliac serology

In this premenopausal woman with no symptoms or relevant history, the priority is to rule out coeliac disease and replace iron as necessary. In this circumstance, menstrual blood loss is presumed to be the cause, as long as anaemia remains non-transfusion dependent. However, it is important to monitor the response to iron therapy, as those that do not have an adequate response may require further investigation.

British Society of Gastroenterology, Guidelines for the management of iron deficiency anaemia, 2011. http://www.bsg.org.uk/images/stories/docs/clinical/guidelines/sbn/bsg_ida_2011.pdf.

21. E. Irradiated red cells

Patients with CLL, particularly those receiving fludarabine, are thought to be at increased risk of transfusion-mediated graft versus host disease (GVHD). For this reason, irradiation of red blood cells is recommended. The reason for the increased incidence of graft versus host disease is that fludarabine is particularly T-cell depleting. Monoclonals which modulate T-cell function such as anti-CD3s may be effective in reducing the incidence of GVHD. Irradiating blood products depletes lymphocytes, including T lymphocytes, which are thought to be a primary driver for GVHD.

Provan D et al., *Oxford Handbook of Clinical Haematology*, Third Edition, Oxford University Press, 2009, Chapter 4, Leukaemia, Chronic lymphocytic leukaemia (B-CLL).

22. A. Acute intermittent porphyria

This presentation is consistent with acute intermittent porphyria which is known as a cause of intermittent abdominal pain, hypertension, hyponatraemia, and agitation. It is frequently misdiagnosed as acute abdomen. Whilst urinary porphyrins are elevated, faecal porphyrins are either normal or very mildly elevated. It occurs due to a mutation in porphobilinogen deaminase. High doses of carbohydrates such as glucose and haematin are the cornerstones of management of acute attacks. Narcotic analgesics may be required for pain relief. Hyponatraemia is mainly due to syndrome of inappropriate antidiuretic hormone secretion (SIADH).

Longmore M et al., *Oxford Handbook of Clinical Medicine*, Eighth Edition, Oxford University Press, 2010, Chapter 15, Clinical chemistry, The porphyrias.

23. B. Hypercalcaemia

Serum potassium is frequently raised following red cell transfusion. The concentration of potassium in blood increases with the length of time the blood is stored (red blood cell membranes deteriorate and allow increasing amounts of potassium to leak from the cells). There have even been case reports of transfusion-associated cardiac arrests, but these tended to be in patients intra-operatively requiring large-volume, rapid transfusions. Red cell transfusions contain a large amount of citrate (~3 g) which acts as an anticoagulant. A healthy adult will hepatically metabolize the citrate within a matter of minutes. However, in the context of massive, rapid transfusion or liver dysfunction the citrate may accumulate. Citrate binds to calcium and can lead to significant hypocalcaemia. Hypercalcaemia is not associated with transfusion. Disturbance of acid–base balance is also seen with massive transfusion. As the blood itself is acidic, patients can initially become acidotic. However, this tends to be reversed, in part due to conversion of citrate and lactate in the blood to bicarbonate by the liver, thus leading to metabolic alkalosis. Thrombocytopaenia may be seen with red cell transfusion due to a dilutional effect, as transfused red cells contain few platelets. Hypothermia may occur if refrigerated blood is given without prior warming.

Smith HM et al., Cardiac arrests associated with hyperkalemia during red blood cell transfusion: a case series, *Anesthesia & Analgesia* 2008;106:1062–1069.

24. C. Transfusion-related lung injury

The history given here is most consistent with non-cardiogenic pulmonary oedema which is associated with transfusion-associated lung injury (TRALI). Chest X-ray usually reveals the presence of multiple nodules. Symptoms are said to begin within six hours of the offending transfused unit. Early involvement of intensivists is crucial, as in other causes of ARDS, with 80% of patients recovering within a few days of onset of the condition.

Benson AB et al., Transfusion-related acute lung injury (TRALI): a clinical review with emphasis on the critically ill, *British Journal of Haematology* 2009;147:437–443. http://onlinelibrary.wiley.com/doi/10.1111/j.1365-2141.2009.07840.x/abstract.

25. A. Bacterial contamination of the platelet unit

Bacterial infection of platelet units is unfortunately quite common, occurring in around 1 in 2000 platelet transfusions. Unlike other blood products, platelets are incubated at 20–40°C before transfusion. As such they are much more at risk of contamination. Early symptoms of fever and rigors are consistent with this clinical picture. Rapid testing of platelet samples has advanced to try and reduce the frequency of platelet contamination, with Gram-positive bacteria such as coagulase-negative *Staphylococci* and *Propionobacterium acnes* being common causes. Checking for blood in the urine is useful as it may be indicative of an acute haemolytic transfusion reaction. The urine should of course also be sent for microscopy, to see if in fact it contains intact red cells, indicating a different diagnosis: bleeding from the urinary tract.

Transfusion Guidelines, Chapter 9: Microbiology tests for donors and donations: general specifications for laboratory test procedures. http://www.transfusionguidelines.org/red-book/chapter-9-microbiology-tests-for-donors-and-donations-general-specifications-for-laboratory-test-procedures.

26. A. t(15;17)

All the above are cytogenetic abnormalities seen in haematological malignancy. The t(15;17) translocation is found in around 95% of cases of acute promyelocytic leukaemia, and leads to production of the PML-RARA fusion protein. t(9;22)(q34;q11) is the Philadelphia translocation, classically associated with chronic myeloid leukaemia, but is also found in acute lymphoblastic leukaemia. The t(8;14) translocation is seen in Burkitt's lymphoma and t(11;14) in Mantle cell lymphoma. Inversion 16 is found in acute myeloid leukaemia.

Warrell DA et al., *Oxford Textbook of Medicine*, Fifth Edition, Oxford University Press, 2010, Section 22.3.4, Acute myeloid leukaemia.

27. A. Lymph node biopsy

Lymph node architecture is associated with prognosis in non-Hodgkin's lymphoma, as such fine needle aspiration biopsy is not recommended versus whole lymph node biopsy for confirming a histological diagnosis. Various scores have been developed for evaluating risk in non-Hodgkin's lymphoma, and contain measures such as number of lymph node sites involved, LDH, age, and functional status. WHO classification exists for evaluating grade of lymphoma from lymph node biopsy. CT chest and abdomen may of course be useful for evaluating the extent of spread of the disease. Staging is according to the Ann Arbor classification: Stage I—a single lymph node area or single extranodal site; Stage II—2 or more lymph node areas on the same side of the diaphragm; Stage III—denotes lymph node areas on both sides of the diaphragm; Stage IV—disseminated or multiple involvement of the extranodal organs. Lymphocyte-rich Hodgkin's on biopsy is associated with the most favourable prognosis.

Provan D et al., *Oxford Handbook of Clinical Haematology*, Third Edition, Oxford University Press, 2009, Chapter 5, Lymphoma Non-Hodgkin lymphoma (NHL).

28. A. IB

The Ann Arbor system is often used to stage Hodgkin's lymphoma, and it influences treatment choice as well as prognosis. The patient undergoes a chest X-ray, CT thorax, abdomen and pelvis, and sometimes a bone marrow biopsy. The numbering of the staging is as follws: stage I—confined to single lymph node region; stage II—involvement of two or more nodal areas on the same side of the diaphragm; stage III—involvement of nodes on both sides of the diaphragm; stage IV—spread beyond the lymph nodes e.g. liver or bone marrow. The 'A' or 'B' depends on the presence of 'B' symptoms. 'A' indicates that there are no systemic symptoms other than pruritus. 'B' indicates that 'B' symptoms are present: weight loss >10% in the last six months, unexplained fever >38°C, or drenching night sweats (requiring change of clothes). This patient therefore falls into the IB bracket.

Longmore M et al., *Oxford Handbook of Clinical Medicine*, Eighth Edition, Oxford University Press, 2010, Chapter 8, Haematology, Hogdkin's lymphoma.

29. B. Inhibition of ADAMTS13

The diagnosis is thrombotic thrombocytopenic purpura, characterized by neurological symptoms, microangiopathic haemolytic anaemia, and thrombocytopenia. There may be renal impairment.

The molecular pathogenesis involves inhibition of ADAMTS13, which prevents cleavage of von Willebrand factor and leads to formation of microthrombi in the circulation. Plasma exchange is the cornerstone of treatment, with steroids or rituximab being used as adjunctive therapy in selected cases. G6PD deficiency results in haemolytic anaemia. Mutations in JAK2 have been identified in patients with myeloproliferative disorders. Acquired C1 esterase inhibitor deficiency leads to a similar condition to hereditary angioedema.

Binder WD et al., Case 37-2010: a 16-year-old girl with confusion, anemia, and thrombocytopenia. *New England Journal of Medicine* 2010;363:2352–61.

30. B. Ciprofloxacin

The features of this scenario are consistent with drug-induced haemolysis against a background of G6PD deficiency which is commoner in patients of Mediterranean or African origin. Symptoms of haemolysis begin 1–3 days after ingestion of the drug and anaemia is most severe 7–10 days after ingestion. Nitrofurantoin, sulphonamides, and quinolones are all recognized to lead to haemolysis in patients with G6PD deficiency, so the correct answer here is ciprofloxacin. Haemolysis is typically self-limiting and is related to the dose of the causative agent used.

Provan D et al., *Oxford Handbook of Clinical Haematology*, Third Edition. Oxford University Press, 2009.

31. C. BCL-2 expression

Prognostic factors in lymphoma are well described, they include: histologic grade; performance status; constitutional ('B') symptoms unfavourable; age (unfavourable >50 years); disseminated disease (stage III–IV) unfavourable; extranodal disease (unfavourable >2 extranodal sites); bulky disease (unfavourable if >10 cm); raised serum LDH raised serum Beta2-microglobulin unfavourable; high proliferation rate by Ki-67 immunochemistry unfavourable; CL-2 expression poor risk in DLBCL (not with R-CHOP treatment); BCL-6 expression favourable in DLBCL (not with R-CHOP treatment); P53 mutations unfavourable; T-cell phenotype unfavourable; high grade transformation from low grade NHL unfavourable; gene expression profile in DLBCL (GCB favourable; ABC poor).

Provan D et al., *Oxford Handbook of Clinical Haematology*, Third Edition, Oxford University Press, 2009.

32. B. Tyrosine kinase inhibitor

Imatinib is a small molecule protein-tyrosine kinase inhibitor that potently inhibits the activity of the Bcr-Abl tyrosine kinase (TK), as well as several receptor TKs: Kit, the receptor for stem cell factor (SCF) coded for by the c-Kit proto-oncogene, the discoidin domain receptors (DDR1 and DDR2), the colony stimulating factor receptor (CSF-1R), and the platelet-derived growth factor receptors alpha and beta (PDGFR-alpha and PDGFR-beta). It is used in the treatment of chronic myeloid leukaemia, a number of myeloproliferative disorders, and in the treatment of gastrointestinal stromal tumours. Histidine kinases are found in plants, fungi, and eukaryotes. Examples of serine kinases include JNK, p38, and MAPK.

Imatinib: summary of product characteristics. http://www.medicines.org.uk/emc/medicine/15014/SPC/GLIVEC%20Tablets#PHARMACODYNAMIC_PROPS.

33. A. Protein S deficiency

Nephrotic syndrome not only leads to loss of albumin into the urine, it leads to the loss of other important proteins such as Protein C and S involved in blood clotting. The correct answer is therefore protein S deficiency. Anti-phospholipid antibody syndrome is most likely to be associated with SLE, we have no reason to believe that the patient should also have Factor V Leiden mutation, and he is more likely to be anaemic than polycythaemic. Potentially lifelong anti-coagulation may be required unless urinary protein excretion can be reduced.

Provan D et al., *Oxford Handbook of Clinical Haematology*, Third Edition, Oxford University Press, 2009.

34. C. Six months

In the absence of precipitating factors, three months' warfarinization is deemed appropriate. In this situation, however, the fact that she is heterozygous for the V Leiden mutation, drives warfarinization for a six-month period. Whether patients are homozygous (very rare), or heterozygous for factor V Leiden, lifelong anti-coagulation is only recommended for two or more thrombotic events. Previously these patients were thought to require life-long warfarinization, although case series now suggest that the benefit risk for life-long versus six months of warfarin therapy is not positive for a first thrombosis. If subsequent events occur then life-long warfarinization may be reconsidered.

Rutherford's *Vascular Surgery*, Eighth Edition, Saunders Elsevier, 2014, Chapter by Cronenwett JL, et al., Hypercoagulable states. http://www.clinicalkey.com.

Kujovich JL, Factor V, Leiden thrombophilia, *Genetics in Medicine* 2011;13:1.

Douketis JD, Deep vein thrombosis, Merck Manual Professional Version. http://www.merckmanuals.com/professional/cardiovascular-disorders/peripheral-venous-disorders/deep-venous-thrombosis-dvt.

35. A. Hereditary spherocytosis

The obvious point here is that whatever has led to her clinical presentation with gallstones and macrocytic anaemia also affected her father. We are not told the results of the blood film, but the suspicion is that she has a raised reticulocyte count and spherocytes, indicating hereditary spherocytosis. In most cases, inheritance follows an autosomal dominant pattern, although autosomal recessive inheritance is also reported. Gallstones are seen in 50% of patients, even in those with relatively mild haemolytic anaemia. Splenectomy is curative, but is reserved for patients >10 years of age.

Provan D et al., *Oxford Handbook of Clinical Haematology*, Third Edition, Oxford University Press, 2009.

36. D. In a patient who has an acute deterioration in renal function

Warfarin is highly protein bound, and it is the unbound component of warfarin which exerts its anticoagulant effect. In patients with acute renal failure the proportion of free versus bound warfarin increases, which leads to increased INR. Carbamazepine and St John's Wort are both enzyme inducers, which leads to a reduction in INR. Chronic stable alcohol consumption also leads to hepatic enzyme induction. Gilbert's syndrome is associated with a defect in bilirubin conjugation, which is not linked to warfarin metabolism.

Warfarin Prescribing Information. http://www.medicines.org.uk/emc/medicine/21562/spc.

37. B. Creatinine 152

To confirm a diagnosis of MGUS, all of the following criteria must be met: serum monoclonal protein <30g/L; bone marrow plasma cells <10% (IgM MGUS—lymphoplasmacytic cells <10%); no evidence of other B-cell lymphoproliferative disorder; no myeloma-related end-organ or tissue impairment, e.g. lytic bone lesions, anaemia, hypercalcaemia, or renal failure (IgM MGUS—no anaemia, constitutional symptoms, hyperviscosity, lymphadenopathy or hepatosplenomegaly).

Provan D et al., *Oxford Handbook of Clinical Haematology*, Third Edition, Oxford University Press, 2009.

38. D. Splenectomy

This patient is suffering from hereditary spherocytosis. He has symptomatic anaemia and is suffering abdominal pain as a result of splenomegaly. Whilst splenectomy is discouraged below the age of 10 years, at this stage it is the most appropriate intervention and is 'curative'. Prior to splenectomy anaemia symptoms may be aleviated with folic acid supplementation. Complications of hereditary spherocytosis are listed below. In this age group haematological malignancy would be considered as a possible cause of splenomegaly, although the fact he is well apart from the anaemia and abdominal pain, and that his sister underwent splenectomy, make this rather unlikely.

Box 2.1 Complications of hereditary spherocytosis

- Aplastic crisis (e.g. parvovirus B19 infection, but may be any virus).
- Megaloblastic changes in folate deficiency.
- ↑ haemolysis during intercurrent illness (e.g. infections).
- Gallstones (in 50% patients; occur even in mild disease).
- Leg ulceration.
- Extramedullary haemopoiesis.
- Fe overload if multiply transfused.

Provan D et al., *Oxford Handbook of Clinical Haematology*, Third Edition, Oxford University Press, 2009.

39. A. Inhibits conversion of plasminogen

Tranexamic acid is an antifibrinolytic compound which is a potent competitive inhibitor of the activation of plasminogen to plasmin. At much higher concentrations it is a non-competitive inhibitor of plasmin. The inhibitory effect of tranexamic acid in plasminogen activation by urokinase has been reported to be 6–100 times and by streptokinase 6–40 times greater than that of aminocaproic acid. Clopidogrel is a platelet ADP receptor inhibitor used as an anti-platelet agent in the prevention of ischaemic cardiovascular disease. Factor Xa inhibitors are proposed as alternative anti-coagulants to warfarin across a range of indications, warfarin is a vitamin K antagonist, and aspirin is a cyclo-oxygenase inhibitor.

Tranexamic acid prescribing information. http://www.medicines.org.uk/emc/medicine/24325.

40. C. Enoxiparin

Guidelines on the management of venous thrombo-embolism in patients with cancer were published in January 2013. They recommend low molecular weight heparin (LMWH) as optimal therapy for VTE in this patient group. Warfarin is best avoided given the presence of a hepatic metastasis and liver dysfunction, as are factor Xa inhibitors for the same reason. Anti-platelet agents are not adequate protection against further VTE events.

Guidelines on VTE in cancer (only read the recommendations that summarize each section): Farge D et al., International clinical practice guidelines for the treatment and prophylaxis of venous thromboembolism in patients with cancer, *Journal of Thrombosis and Haemostasis* 2013;11:36–57. http://www.ncbi.nlm.nih.gov/pubmed/23217107.

41. D. Discontinue dosing for a few days and give vitamin K 5 mg IV

Guidelines suggest that even in the absence of active bleeding, an INR>8 necessitates at least partial reversal of warfarin, with 5 mg IV vitamin K. For INRs between 5 and 8, if there is no active bleeding, warfarin may be omitted without the need for additional therapy. For any major bleeding episode where INR is elevated, both vitamin K and prothrombin complex concentrate should be given. Minor bleeding episodes at INRs of <8 can be managed with smaller doses of IV vitamin K.

British Society of clinical haematology guidelines. http://www.bcshguidelines.com/documents/warfarin_4th_ed.pdf.

42. B. Give low molecular weight heparin and suggest she returns for an ultrasound

NICE guidelines recommend that any patient with suspected venous thromboembolic disease should be given anti-coagulation if they are to wait more than four hours for a definitive investigation. This is now established as a quality standard. As such she should be given low molecular weight heparin and return the morning afterwards for a venous ultrasound.

NICE guidelines on management of venous thromboembolism. https://www.nice.org.uk/guidance/qs29.

43. B. JAK2 mutation

JAK2 is a non receptor tyrosine kinase. Mutations in JAK2 have been implicated in the development of a range of myeloproliferative disorders, including primary polycythaemia, essential thrombocythaemia and myelofibrosis. Affordable and practical genetic testing for JAK2 is currently under development. Levels of erythropoeitin and ferritin are often low in patients with primary polycythaemia. The Philadelphia translocation is most associated with chronic myeloid leukaemia.

Warrell DA et al., *Oxford Textbook of Medicine*, Fifth Edition, Oxford University Press, 2010, Chapter 22.3.8 The polycythaemias.

44. C. Add phlebotomy

This man is at very high risk of suffering a stroke. As such rapid intervention to reduce his haematocrit/viscosity is therefore required as well as starting aspirin therapy. Out of the options given, hydroxycarbamide is definitely indicated, although the quickest way to reduce his haematocrit is by venesection. Other options apart from hydroxycarbamide for inducing myelosuppression include hydroxyurea, interferon alpha, and ruxolitinib, a specific JAK inhibitor although this is not currently recommended by NICE. In the setting of a normal haematocrit post venesection/myelosuppression, further anti-platelet therapy with clopidogrel may be indicated, but not at the current time.

Warrell DA et al., *Oxford Textbook of Medicine*, Fifth Edition, Oxford University Press, 2010: The polycythaemias.

45. C. Full spinal MRI scan

Metastatic spinal cord compression in an oncological emergency. NICE have produced guidelines for the management of this condition. They recommend that an MRI of the whole spine is carried out as soon as possible to diagnose this condition and to plan the most appropriate treatment. X-rays and CT scans do not give accurate enough images of the spinal cord to diagnose this problem. PSA and prostate biopsy may help in the diagnosis and monitoring of prostate cancer, but the most pressing concern here is spinal cord compression, and this needs to be looked into more urgently. The reference here describing the NICE guidance for this condition is useful.

NICE Guidance on Metastatic Spinal Cord Compression. http://pathways.nice.org.uk/pathways/metastatic-spinal-cord-compression.

46. E. Extrathoracic lymph node biopsy

This is a case of superior vena cava obstruction. Differential diagnoses include primary lung malignancy (especially small cell), lymphoma (most likely in this patient), and, rarely, non-malignant causes (e.g. goitre). Unless there is evidence of stridor or laryngeal oedema, a definitive diagnosis should be sought before treatment is commenced. Prior radiotherapy can interfere with histological diagnosis and steroids make lymphoma more difficult to diagnose. Tissue diagnosis is the gold standard. Bronchoscopy is associated with a high risk of bleeding post-biopsy due to venous congestion.

Wan JF, Bezjak A, Superior vena cava syndrome, *Hematology/Oncology Clinics of North America* 2010;24(3): 501–513.

47. D. Higher socio-economic status is associated with a greater risk of breast cancer

Prolonged exposure to unopposed endogenous oestrogens most strongly influences breast cancer risk. Hence early menarche and late menopause are associated with an increased incidence of breast cancer whilst age at first live birth, parity, and breastfeeding also appear to influence risk. Males with Klinefelter's syndrome (XXY) demonstrate a marked increase in breast cancer risk, compared to the normal male population, with one study suggesting this may be as high as 50-fold. Many studies have investigated the potential effects of alcohol on breast cancer risk. Consumption of as few as one or two alcoholic drinks per day appears to be associated with a higher risk, and multiple studies have found a consistent association between greater intake (>2 units/day) and increased incidence of hormone receptor-positive breast cancers. Various mechanisms have been proposed including increased exposure to circulating oestrogens and androgens, and increased rates of DNA damage. Higher socio-economic status is also associated with a greater risk of breast cancer. However this is not believed to be an independent risk factor. Rather it reflects differences in lifestyle, including age at first birth, participation in screening programmes, etc. Women who have inherited a mutation of the *BRCA1* or *BRCA2* gene have up to an 87% lifetime risk of developing breast cancer.

Cassidy J et al., *Oxford Handbook of Oncology*, Third Edition, Oxford University Press, 2010, Chapter 15, Breast cancer.

48. C. BCAR4

BCAR-4 is a key gene thought to drive resistance to anti-oestrogens such as tamoxifen. In studies it is associated with both decreased metastasis-free survival and mortality representing increased tumour aggressiveness. This resistance is thought to be mediated via ERBB2/ERBB3 signalling, the activity of which is significantly increased in BCAR4-positive tumour cells. It is thought that eventually BCAR4 typing may impact on choices for adjuvant therapy for breast cancer on top of surgery alone.

Godinho MFE et al., Relevance of BCAR4 in tamoxifen resistance and tumour aggressiveness of human breast cancer, *British Journal of Cancer* 2010;103:1284–1291. http://www.nature.com/bjc/journal/v103/n8/full/6605884a.html.

49. D. Treatment is usually with urgent rehydration, followed by bisphosphonates

Malignant hypercalcaemia is observed in up to 30% of patients with solid tumours and leukaemias at some stage in their illness and is usually associated with advanced disease, in particular breast and prostate cancer, myeloma, lymphoma, and squamous cell carcinoma of the lung. However, it is an uncommon mode of presentation of previously undiagnosed malignancy. Although osteolysis induced by lytic skeletal metastases is a recognized mechanism, hypercalcaemia can be seen even in the absence of overt boney involvement. For instance, it may be mediated by humoral factors, such as parathyroid hormone-related peptide (PTHrP), a humoral factor seen particularly in squamous cell carcinoma of the lung and non-Hodgkin's lymphoma known to mediate hypercalcaemia. Presentation may be acute or insidious. In patients presenting acutely with hypercalcaemia, the calcium acts as a powerful diuretic, causing renal loss of both salt and water. Dehydration and subsequent pre-renal renal failure may be marked and rehydration is the priority. Indeed rehydration with 0.9% normal saline may be sufficient to return the serum calcium to the normal range. Administration of bisphosphonates to cause inhibition of osteoclast activity can be considered once renal function is adequate. However, it is not effective until around 48 hours after administration and therefore is not used in the initial resuscitation. Steroids have little role in the management of hypercalcaemia associated with solid tumours, although they can be used in haematological malignancies such as myeloma. Limiting dietary intake of calcium is almost never helpful. Chvostek's sign is typical of hypocalcaemia.

Cassidy J et al., *Oxford Handbook of Oncology*, Third Edition, Oxford University Press, 2010, Chapter 36, Biochemical crises.

50. A. Testicular cancer accounts for only around 1% of cancers in men

Testicular cancer does account for only 1% of cancers in men, although it remains the most common cancer affecting young men (15–35 years old). 95% of testicular cancers are germ cell tumours, either seminomas (55%) or non-seminomatous tumours such as teratomas. Ten per cent of cases are in patients with a history of undescended testes, with a quarter of these occurring in the contralateral normally descended side. Although haemorrhage or infarction secondary to the cancer may present with pain, acute pain is a presenting feature in only around 10% of such cancers. Most commonly, testicular malignancy presents as painless swelling of one testicle or sometimes as a heaviness or ache in the groin or lower abdomen. Symptoms attributable to metastatic disease are observed at presentation in around 10% of patients, which may include neck masses, respiratory symptoms such as cough or dyspnoea, back pain, and central and/or peripheral neurological symptoms. Only around 5% of men with testicular germ cell tumours present with gynaecomastia, usually associated with foci of choriocarcinoma or trophoblastic cells within the tumour and typically, although not exclusively, attributed to production of high levels of hCG. Structural similarities between TSH and hCG result in hCG possessing weak thyroid stimulating activity. Consequently, paraneoplastic hyperthyroidism may be observed in patients presenting with testicular cancer. Specific treatment for hyperthyroidism is not indicated; treatment should instead be aimed at the underlying malignant disease.

Krege S et al., European Consensus conference on diagnosis and treatment of germ cell cancer: a report of the second meeting of the European Germ Cell Cancer Consensus group (EGCCCG): part I, *European Urology* 2008;53(3):478–496.

51. D. Excision biopsy of a lymph node

Two of the most important factors with respect to determining prognosis in lymphoma include lymph node architecture, and abnormal lymph nodes above and below the diaphragm. As such out of the options given, it is excision of a lymph node with biopsy that will give most information. Whilst PET scanning of the head and neck will offer information about which lymph nodes are abnormal, it won't be as useful as excision biopsy of a node. FNA will yield abnormal cells, but not help with determining architecture. Bone marrow examination is an important part of the diagnostic work-up, but at this stage is less useful with respect to prognosis than lymph node excision. Whilst peripheral blood cytogenetics may yield abnormal cells, again this has much less utility than the correct option. Low-grade non-Hodgkin's lymphoma is associated with a good prognosis, with median survival now approaching 10 years.

Provan D et al., *Oxford Handbook of Clinical Haematology*, Third Edition, Oxford University Press, 2009.

CARDIOLOGY

QUESTIONS

3

1. **A 20-year-old man with a history of illicit drug abuse was admitted with endocarditis. The echocardiogram revealed large vegetations. Which of the following organisms is the most frequent causative agent?**
   A. Staphylococcus aureus
   B. Streptococcus bovis
   C. Streptococcus sanguis
   D. Staphylococcus epidermidis
   E. Streptococcal pneumonia

2. **The following are not signs of severe aortic regurgitation:**
   A. Breathlessness on mild exertion
   B. Dilated heart clinically
   C. Long diastolic murmur
   D. Low diastolic blood pressure
   E. Resting tachycardia

3. **A 40-year-old woman comes to the clinic for the results of her 72 h Holter monitor. She has complained of palpitations on a number of occasions over the past few months, but she finds these difficult to describe and they are not associated with significant symptoms of syncope or pre-syncope, or any change in her exercise capacity. There is no other relevant past medical history. On examination her BP is 110/70, her pulse is 70 and regular. Her Holter was normal apart from one period where five PVEs occured in one minute. How would you manage this woman?**
   A. Arrange an angiogram
   B. Start amiodarone
   C. Reassure her
   D. Start a beta blocker
   E. Start a non-dihydropyridine calcium antagonist

4. **Which of the following is not a conventional risk factor for sudden cardiac death taken into account when deciding to implant an implantable cardioverter defibrillator (ICD) as primary prophylaxis in hypertrophic cardiomyopathy?**
    A. Abnormal blood pressure response to exercise
    B. Family history of sudden cardiac death
    C. Gadolimium enhancement on cardiac magnetic resonance imaging
    D. Maximal left ventricular wall thickness > 30 mm
    E. Non-sustained ventricular tachycardia on Holter monitoring

5. **A 24-year-old man is successfully resuscitated after a cardiac arrest whilst playing football for his local pub team. On follow-up examination in the cardiology clinic he is noted to have a BP of 145/85. There is a double apical impulse and ejection systolic murmur. On reviewing his notes you see that he had a number of episodes of non-sustained VT whilst being monitored on the coronary care unit. Which of the following is the intervention most likely to prolong his life?**
    A. Amiodarone
    B. Permanent pacing
    C. Implantable cardioverter defibrillator
    D. Surgical Myomectomy
    E. Alcohol septal ablation

6. **A 61-year-old man is diagnosed with subacute bacterial endocarditis. He has refused to visit the dentist for many years and over the past few weeks has suffered from increasing lethargy, anorexia, and night sweats. On examination his BP is 144/79, his temperature is 37.8°C, and his pulse is 74 and regular. He has a pan-systolic murmur loudest in the mitral area. Investigations: Hb 10.4, WCC 12.5, PLT 210, Na 137, K 4.9, Cr 110, ESR 92, ECG—PR interval 175 ms, ECHO—Multiple mitral valve vegetations. Which of the following is an indication for urgent surgery after 14 days of antibiotic therapy?**
    A. Rising ESR
    B. Failure of fever to settle
    C. Enlarging vegetations
    D. Lenghtening PR interval
    E. Persistent murmur

7. **Which of the following enzymes rises the latest after a myocardial infarction?**
    A. Glucose phosphate isoenzyme BB (GPBB)
    B. ALT
    C. CK
    D. LDH
    E. Troponin I

8. **A 64-year-old woman comes to the cardiology clinic for review. She has two failed electrical cardioversions and is now deemed to have permanent atrial fibrillation. There is little other significant past medical history apart from a previous inferior myocardial infarction. On examination her BP is 146/83, pulse is 85 atrial fibrillation. Echocardiography reveals moderate left atrial enlargement. Which of the following is the correct advice with respect to anti-platelet/anti-coagulation therapy?**

   A. Aspirin 75 mg

   B. Aspirin 300 mg

   C. Aspirin 75 mg and clopidogrel 75 mg

   D. Clopidogrel 75 mg

   E. Warfarin

9. **A 62-year-old woman with a history of diabetes mellitus and smoking 20 cigarettes per day comes to the clinic for review. Her BP is noted to be 145/81 and she has reversed splitting of the second heart sound. There are bilateral basal crackles on auscultation of the chest. Investigations: Hb 12.1 g/dl, WCC 8.0 x10^9/l, PLT 199 x10^9/l, Na$^+$ 137 mmol/l, K$^+$ 4.2 mmol/l, creatinine 143 micromol/l. Which of the following is the most likely cause of reversed splitting of the second heart sound?**

   A. ASD

   B. Aortic regurgitation

   C. Left bundle branch block

   D. Right bundle branch block

   E. Mitral regurgitation

10. **A 67-year-old man with a long history of ischaemic heart disease presents to the emergency department with rapid palpitations and feelings of light headedness. On examination his BP is 135/80; his ventricular rate is above 180 on the monitor. There are bilateral crackles on auscultation of the chest and mild ankle swelling. ECG—Monomorphic ventricular tachycardia, K$^+$ 4.2, Mg^{2+} 0.85. Which of the following is the most appropriate next treatment step?**

    A. Urgent DC cardioversion

    B. Amiodarone and magnesium

    C. Amiodarone and potassium

    D. Amiodarone

    E. Sotolol

11. **A 57-year-old man with a history of smoking, hypertension, and Type 2 diabetes managed with metformin presents to the emergency department with two hours of central chest pain, nausea, and sweating. On examination his BP is 110/60, he looks grey and sweaty. His pulse is 90 and regular. He is not in cardiac failure and is currently pain free. His ECG reveals inferolateral ST depression. He has been given aspirin and GTN by the nursing staff. Which of the following is the next appropriate therapy?**

A. Clopidogrel 75 mg
B. Clopidogrel 300 mg
C. GTN infusion
D. Diamorphine
E. LMW herparin

12. **A patient who is pregnant develops high blood pressure which requires treatment. Which of these medications should be avoided if at all possible?**

A. Methyldopa
B. Nifedipine
C. Ramipril
D. Hydralazine
E. Labetolol

13. **A 28-year-old marathon runner comes to the emergency room for review. She ran a half marathon a few days earlier, despite the fact that she was suffering from symptoms of a cold, and now has shortness of breath and is unable to exercise. On examination her BP is 90/50 and her pulse is 90 and regular. She has bilateral crackles and mild ankle swelling. You suspect myocarditis. Which of the following is the most likely cause?**

A. Epstein–Barr virus
B. Coxsackie virus
C. Influenza A
D. Influenza B
E. Adenovirus

14. **The diagnosis of constrictive pericarditis is more likely than restrictive cardiomyopathy if:**

A. Tissue Doppler confirms a peak early velocity of longitudinal expansion (Ea) of less than 8 cm s^{-1}
B. Cardiac catheterization confirms a difference of more than 6 mmHg between the right and left end diastolic pressures
C. Cardiac catheterization confirms the pulmonary artery pressure is greater than 50 mmHg
D. Imaging confirms pericardial calcification
E. Strain imaging confirms reduced myocardial systolic contractility

15. **Carney syndrome is associated with:**
    A. Incomplete penetrance
    B. Autosomal recessive inheritance
    C. *PRKAR1A* gene mutations
    D. *CK* transporter gene mutations
    E. Genetic anticipation

16. **A 24-year-old man presents with a history of recurrent seizures at night. There is a family history of a brother having died suddenly at the age of 15 with no cause of death having been established. In the course of investigation he has the following ECG performed. What is the most likely diagnosis? (See Figure 3.1)**
    A. Brugada syndrome
    B. Catecholaminergic polymorphic ventricular tachycardia (CPVT)
    C. Congenital long QT syndrome, type 2
    D. Right ventricular dysplasia
    E. Atrioventricular septation defect—AVSD (previously known as ostium primum ASD)

17. **A 17-year-old woman presents with palpitations and dizziness. She reports a few short-lived palpitations in the past but nothing this severe. Her ECG is as shown in Figure 3.2. What is the best description of her arrhythmia?**
    A. Atrial fibrillation with rate-related aberration
    B. Polymorphic ventricular tachycardia
    C. Pre-excited atrial fibrillation
    D. Right ventricular outflow tract tachycardia
    E. Ventricular tachycardia with capture beats

18. **A 55-year-old man presents two weeks post discharge having had a myocardial infarction complaining of orthopnoea and NYHA grade III shortness of breath on exertion. He is taking 10 mg of bisoprolol and 5 mg of ramipril. His heart rate is 70 and BP 120/70. ECG shows left bundle branch block and CXR is congested. An echo shows an ejection fraction of 30%. The most appropriate prognostic intervention is:**
    A. Add an angiotensin receptor antagonist
    B. Biventricular pacing
    C. Digoxin
    D. Eplerenone
    E. Ivabradine

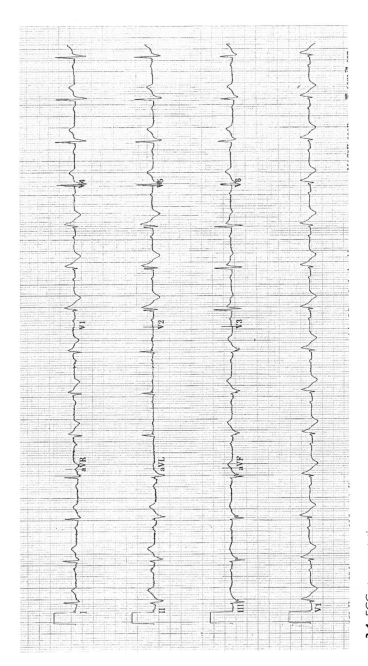

Figure 3.1 ECG at presentation

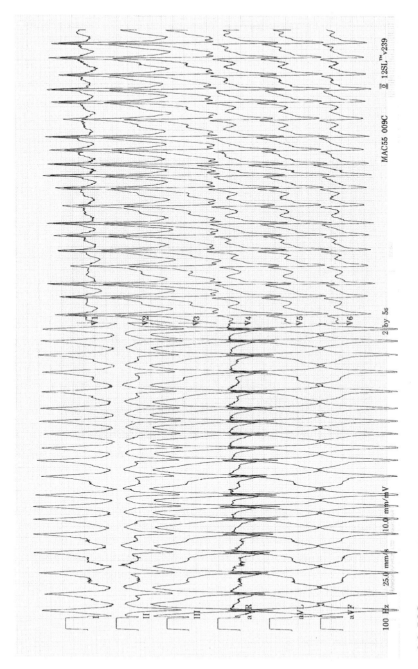

Figure 3.2 ECG at presentation

19. **A 50-year-old man presents with a history of a collapse without loss of consciousness. On examination his blood pressure is 165/95 mmHg and he has a quiet systolic murmur. His examination is otherwise normal. Transthoracic echocardiography was performed and the M mode tracing shown in Figure 3.3 was taken. What is the most likely diagnosis?**

    A. Amyloidosis
    B. Fabry's disease
    C. Hypertrophic cardiomyopathy
    D. Kearns–Sayres syndrome
    E. Left ventricular hypertrophy

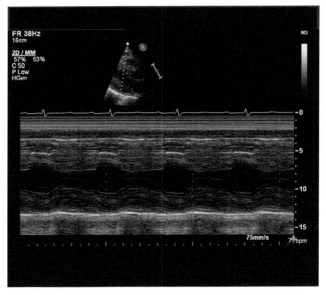

Figure 3.3 M mode trace taken across the left ventricle

20. **A 75-year-old hypertensive man presents with mild breathlessness on exertion. There is no other relevant past medical history. Physical examination reveals atrial fibrillation at a rate of 100, but is otherwise unremarkable. Routine investigations, including thyroid function tests, are normal. Echo shows a dilated left atrium and mild to moderately impaired left ventricular function. The most appropriate initial medical management is:**

    A. Beta blocker and aspirin
    B. Beta blocker and warfarin
    C. Digoxin and aspirin
    D. Digoxin and warfarin.
    E. Furosemide and warfarin

21. **A 68-year-old woman is referred to you with an established diagnosis of stable angina. She is on aspirin, the maximum dose of a beta blocker and nitrate that she can tolerate and is known to have single vessel coronary disease in the right coronary artery. On examination pulse is 65, BP 135/85, and there are no abnormal findings. The best form of therapy to manage her symptoms would be:**
    A. ACE inhibitor
    B. Coronary artery bypass grafting
    C. Dihydropyridine calcium antagonist
    D. Ivabradine
    E. Percutaneous coronary intervention

22. **A 57-year-old man presents with a one-year history of angina which limits him at approximately 200 m. Angiography shows a 90% stenosis in his right coronary artery. Which of the following treatments will have the most positive impact on his prognosis?**
    A. Amlodipine
    B. Furosermide
    C. Isosorbide mononitrate
    D. Lisinopril
    E. Percutaneous coronary internvention

23. **Which of the following statements is true regarding rheumatic valvular heart disease?**
    A. Erythema nodosum is one of the major criteria for the diagnosis of rheumatic fever
    B. Rheumatic fever is now a rare condition worldwide
    C. Symptons due to valvular involvement usually start within months of the episode of rheumatic fever
    D. The condition occurs as a result of carditis caused by a group D streptococcus
    E. The tips of the valves are preferentially affected by the inflammatory process

24. **A 48-year-old woman presents with no cardiac risk factors and central chest pain that sometimes occurs on exertion. The most appropriate diagnostic investigation would be:**
    A. Cardiac stress MRI
    B. Coronary calcium score
    C. CXR
    D. Exercise ECG
    E. MIBI prefusion scan

25. **Which of the following is not a feature of a vulnerable (unstable) atherosclerotic plaque?**

    A. Abundant neutrophils
    B. Frequent apoptotic smooth muscle cells
    C. Large lipid core
    D. Low collagen content in the cap
    E. Thin fibrous cap

26. **A 50-year-old man is referred for further management of hypertension. He has no other past medical history and specifically no lung disease. He is taking ramipril 10 mg od and bendroflumethiazide 2.5 mg daily. On examination his blood pressure is 140/90 mmHg and his GP has obtained very similar readings on two previous occasions. Investigations: Electrolytes: potassium 4.8 mmol. ECG: voltage criteria for left ventricular hypertrophy. What is the most appropriate additional medication?**

    A. Alpha blocker
    B. Beta blocker
    C. Dihydopyridine calcium antagonist
    D. No additional medication is needed
    E. Spironolactone

27. **A 57-year-old woman presents with a three-month history of worsening exertional dyspnoea. Investigations: chest X-ray: globular cardiomegaly. Echocardiography: normal cardiac function, global pericardial effusion with evidence of tamponade. What is the most likely physical finding to be present in this situation?**

    A. Extension of the area of cardiac dullness beyond the position of the apex beat
    B. Pericardial rub
    C. Signs of pulmonary oedema
    D. Steep y descent of the jugular venous pulse
    E. Tachycardia

28. **A 45-year-old man presents to the emergency room with an episode of fast irregular palpitations. He works as a publican and admits to significant excess consumption of alcohol. On examination he has an irregular pulse of 120 bpm, and a blood pressure of 110/60 mmHg. Auscultation of his chest reveals bilateral crackles. Echocardiography demonstrates biventricular dilatation with global hypokinesia. Which of the following is likely to have the greatest impact on his long-term prognosis?**
    A. Carvedilol
    B. Cessation of alcohol
    C. Furosemide
    D. Ramipril
    E. Spironolactone

29. **The diagnosis of constrictive pericarditis is more likely than restrictive cardiomyopathy if:**
    A. Tissue Doppler confirms a peak early velocity of longitudinal expansion (Ea) of less than 8 cm s^{-1}
    B. Cardiac catheterization confirms a difference of more than 6 mmHg between the right and left end diastolic pressures
    C. Cardiac catheterization confirms the pulmonary artery pressure is greater than 50 mmHg
    D. Imaging confirms pericardial calcification
    E. Strain imaging confirms reduced myocardial systolic contractility

30. **In patients with atrial septal defects:**
    A. Intracardiac shunting decreases with age due to progressive atrial adhesion and scarring
    B. Intracardiac shunting increases with age due to increasing left ventricular stiffness
    C. Procedural risks of closure outweigh benefits in symptomatic patients over 65 years of age
    D. Sinus venosus defects are more amenable to transcatheter closure than secundum defects
    E. Endocarditis is not uncommon and antibiotic prophylaxis is recommended

31. A 53-year-old woman presents with shortness of breath, orthopnoea, and paroxysmal nocturnal dyspnoea. She has had a history of rheumatoid arthritis since the age of 24 and has been treated with multiple medications but is currently taking sulfasalazine, methotrexate, and ibuprofen. On examination her rheumatoid arthritis is relatively quiescent. Her pulse is regular at 88 bpm and her blood pressure is 140/85 mmHg. Her jugular venous pressure is elevated 5 cm above the sternal angle of Louis and she has bilateral basal crepitations. Investigations: Full blood count: Haemoglobin 10.9 g/dl; Liver function tests: Serum globulin 43 g/l, serum albumin 27 g/l; Urinalysis: Blood –ve, protein 2+, nitrite –ve, leucocytes –ve. What is the most likely diagnosis?

    A. Amyloidosis
    B. Dilated cardiomyopathy
    C. Haemochromatosis
    D. Hypertrophic cardiomyopathy
    E. Libman–Sacks endocarditis

32. A 68-year-old man has failed two cardioversions for atrial fibrillation. He is known to have ischaemic heart disease and has left atrial enlargement and LV dysfunction. He takes lisinopril, furosemide, aspirin, and simvastatin. On examination his BP is 142/82, his pulse is 91 atrial fibrillation. There are bilateral crackles at both lung bases. Full blood count and U&E are normal. Which of the following is the optimal choice with respect to rate control?

    A. Digoxin
    B. Amiodarone
    C. Diltiazem
    D. Bisoprolol
    E. Verapamil

33. A 56-year-old man is admitted with severe tightness across his chest lasting 1.5 hours. Clinical examination reveals a distressed patient with sinus tachycardia and blood pressure 170/95 mmHg. There are no signs of cardiac failure and the examination is otherwise unremarkable. His ECG shows changes consistent with acute inferior myocardial infarct. Three days later he develops severe shortness of breath and you are asked to see him. He has bilateral basal crepitations and a systolic heart murmur. What is the cause of his deterioration?

    A. Cardiogenic shock
    B. Further myocardial infarct
    C. Pericarditis
    D. Ruptured chordae tendinae
    E. Tamponade

34. **Restrictive cardiomyopathy is associated with all of the following except:**
    A. Scleroderma
    B. Myotonic dystrophy
    C. Sarcoidosis
    D. Haemochromatosis
    E. Fabry's disease

35. **Indications for revision surgery after mitral valve repair include all of the following except:**
    A. Persistent mitral regurgitation grade 2+
    B. Persistent LVOT obstruction
    C. Mitral stenosis (mean gradient ≥6 mmHg, MVA <1.5 cm²)
    D. Leaflet perforation
    E. Persistent left ventricular dilation

36. **Ankylosing spondylitis:**
    A. Affects approximately 50% of HLA-B27-positive individuals
    B. Is more common among females
    C. Is associated with scarring and constriction of the ascending aorta
    D. Is more commonly associated with aortic regurgitation than mitral regurgitation
    E. Is frequently associated with early onset coronary atherosclerosis

37. **Brugada syndrome is:**
    A. Transmitted in an autosomal recessive pattern
    B. Caused by KCNJ2 mutations encoding inward rectifying K+ channel Kir2.1
    C. Associated with LBBB and ST elevation in V1-3
    D. Treatable with procainamide or ajmaline
    E. Not an indication for beta-blocker therapy

38. **The largest contributor to mortality in Ehlers–Danlos Syndrome type IV is:**
    A. Cardiac failure secondary to mitral regurgitation
    B. Spontaneous arterial rupture
    C. Spontaneous intestinal rupture
    D. Uncontrolled bleeding following external injury
    E. Infections due to immunosuppression and impaired healing

39. **In the United Kingdom, aortic stenosis requiring surgery is most commonly due to:**
    A. Calcific degeneration of a tricuspid valve
    B. Calcific degeneration of a bicuspid valve
    C. Calcific degeneration of a unicuspid valve
    D. Rheumatic degeneration of a tricuspid valve
    E. Metabolic derangements (hypercalcaemia and hyperuricaemia)

40. **The ECG in Figure 3.4 was recorded from a patient admitted with chest pain. A diagnosis of ventricular tachycardia was made. Where in the heart is this arrhythmia likely to have originated?**

    A. Left ventricular apex
    B. Left ventricular free wall
    C. Left ventricular outflow tract
    D. Right ventricular apex
    E. Right ventricular outflow tract

41. **A 38-year-old man is seen in the cardiology clinic following an 18-month history of progressive exertional dyspnoea and fatigue. He was found to have a grade 4/6 systolic murmur at the left sternal edge. ECG showed atrial fibrillation with a heart rate of 104 bpm. Echocardiogram has confirmed a diagnosis HOCM, with a septal wall thickness of 2.6 cm. Which of the following is the best way to manage his symptoms?**

    A. Bisoprolol
    B. Myomectomy
    C. Implantable cardioverter defibrillator
    D. Digoxin
    E. Ramipril

42. **Intravenous adenosine is unlikely to be useful in terminating which of the following arrhythmias?**

    A. Atrial flutter with 2:1 atrioventricular block
    B. Atrioventricular nodal re-entry tachycardia
    C. Catecholamine-sensitive ventricular tachycardia
    D. Sinus node re-entry tachycardia
    E. Orthodromic atrioventricular re-entry tachycardia

43. **Which one of the following features is true of atrial septal defects (ASD)?**

    A. Reversed splitting of the second heart sound is invariable
    B. Sinus venosus defects may occur near the orifice of the inferior vena cava
    C. Secundum type defects are anatomically analogous to a patent foramen ovale
    D. Secundum type defects occur commonly in patients with Down's syndrome
    E. The ECG shows right bundle branch block with left axis deviation in secundum type defects

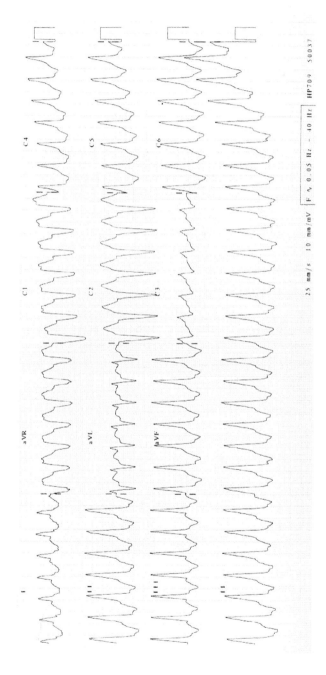

Figure 3.4 ECG demonstrating ventricular tachycardia originating from the right ventricular outflow tract

44. **A 70-year-old man presents with aortic valve infective endocarditis. Regarding indications for surgery for native valve endocarditis, according to the European Society of Cardiology guidelines, which of the following scenarios carries the highest level of evidence?**
   A. Infective endocarditis with co-existing severe coronary disease
   B. Patients with left-sided infective endocarditis and severe regurgitation without heart failure
   C. Patients with infective endocarditis complicated by locally uncontrolled infection, e.g. abscess formation
   D. Patients with vegetations >10 mm and signs of heart failure
   E. Patients with very large vegetations (in excess of 15 mm)

45. **A 22-year-old asymptomatic man has an ECG recorded after the sudden death of a sibling. His ECG shows an epsilon wave in V1. What is the most likely diagnosis?**
   A. Hypertrophic cardiomyopathy
   B. Dilated cardiomyopathy
   C. Arrhythmogenic right ventricular cardiomyopathy
   D. Brugada syndrome
   E. Normal variant

46. **An 18-year-old Caucasian woman is successfully resuscitated after suffering a cardiac arrest during swimming. She has no past medical history, but her brother died suddenly at 14 years of age, also during swimming. Following resuscitation and recovery, she has an echocardiogram which shows a structurally normal heart. What is the most likely diagnosis?**
   A. Brugada syndrome
   B. Dilated cardiomyopathy
   C. Hypertrophic cardiomyopathy
   D. Long QT syndrome type 1
   E. Long QT syndrome type 2

47. **A 23-year-old man was admitted with a one-month history of lethargy, weight loss, and night-sweats. His past medical history included intravenous drug abuse for the preceding two years. On examination he had a soft systolic murmur. Echocardiography demonstrated large vegetations on his tricuspid valve. Fungal endocarditis was suspected but fungal serology was negative. What is the most likely diagnosis?**
   A. Fungal endocarditis is less common in patients with prosthetic valves than those with normal native valves
   B. Fungal endocarditis is rarely associated with bulky valvular vegetations
   C. Fungal endocarditis is unlikely in the absence of positive fungal serology
   D. The mortality rate of fungal endocarditis is up to 15%
   E. The most common organism in fungal endocarditis is Candida species

48. **An 82-year-old man became acutely short of breath and very distressed on a cardiology ward. He had been admitted three days earlier with a late presentation of an inferior myocardial infarction which was managed conservatively. On examination he was pale and sweaty and in obvious distress. He had a regular pulse of 105 bpm and a blood pressure of 122/72 mmHg. He had a loud pan-systolic murmur. Which of the following is the most likely diagnosis?**
    A. Acute mitral valve rupture
    B. Ventricular septal rupture
    C. Ventricular free wall rupture
    D. Cardiac tamponade
    E. Aortic dissection

49. **A 67-year-old man was admitted 10 days after discharge from hospital (following an acute inferior myocardial infarct) with pleuritic chest pain. His d-dimer and troponin levels are normal and a nuclear lung scan showed no evidence of a pulmonary embolism. His haemoglobin is 12.9 g/dl and ESR 56 mm/hour. ECG is identical to the last ECG taken when he was an inpatient with his myocardial infarct. Urea, electrolytes, liver function tests, and corrected calcium are normal. What is the likely cause of his pain?**
    A. Aortic dissection
    B. Cardiac neurosis
    C. Dressler's syndrome
    D. Pneumonia
    E. Recurrent myocardial infarction

50. **Which of the following is a European class I indication for permanent pacemaker implantation?**
    A. Complete atrio-ventricular block two days following elective mitral valve replacement
    B. Mobitz II second-degree heart block day one post right coronary artery territory myocardial infarction
    C. Myotonic dystrophy with second-degree heart block.
    D. Recurrent pre-syncope associated with carotid sinus pressure, associated with a two-second ventricular pause on formal carotid sinus massage
    E. Symptomatic spontaneous sinus bradycardia at a rate of 50 bpm

51. **A 63-year-old woman was admitted with exertional dyspnoea
    18 months after treatment for a left-sided breast cancer. Her
    physical examination was unremarkable apart from a scar
    from left breast surgery. Her chest X-ray showed an increase in
    cardiothoracic ratio and a pericardial effusion was confirmed on
    echocardiography. What is the most appropriate management?**

    A. CT pulmonary angiography to exclude pulmonary emboli as the cause of her dyspnoea
    B. Coronary angiography to exclude angina as a cause of her dyspnoea
    C. High-resolution CT scan of lungs to exclude radiation-induced pulmonary fibrosis as a
       cause of dyspnoea
    D. Percutaneous drainage of the pericardial effusion
    E. Reassure and repeat echocardiography in three months

52. **A 60-year-old Caucasian man presents to casualty on a Monday morning
    complaining of a two-day history of chest pain. He has a history of
    hypertension and is a non-smoker. He is not diabetic. There is no
    relevant family history. His ECG is shown in Figure 3.5. Which initial
    investigation is most appropriate to confirm the diagnosis?**

    A. Cardiac magnetic resonance (CMR) scan
    B. Coronary angiogram
    C. Measurement of cardiac troponin levels
    D. Thoracic computed tomography (CT) scan
    E. Transthoracic echocardiogram

53. **A 61-year-old man is admitted with an infective exacerbation of
    COPD. His BP is noted to be persistently 200/140 mmHg. Review
    is made of a CT abdomen and pelvis that he underwent three
    months earlier to exclude an aortic aneurysm. Which of these CT
    findings is least likely to relate to his elevated blood pressure?**

    A. The left kidney being much smaller than the right
    B. Splenomegaly
    C. Marked calcification of the abdominal aorta
    D. A 2 cm enhancing soft tissue mass arising from the right adrenal gland
    E. Numerous renal, liver, and pancreatic cysts

54. **A 25-year-old man with cystic fibrosis and a history of recurrent chest
    infections was admitted to hospital complaining of recurrent light-
    headedness. He has recently been treated for bronchiectasis by his GP.
    An ECG was performed which is shown in Figure 3.6. Which medication
    is most likely to be responsible for his symptoms?**

    A. Carbocisteine
    B. Clarithromycin
    C. Co-amoxiclav
    D. Ethambutol
    E. Rifampicin

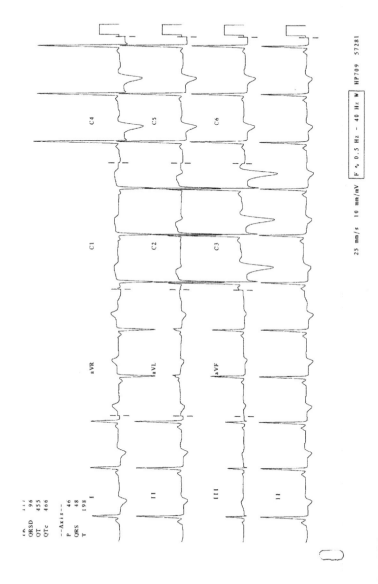

Figure 3.5 ECG

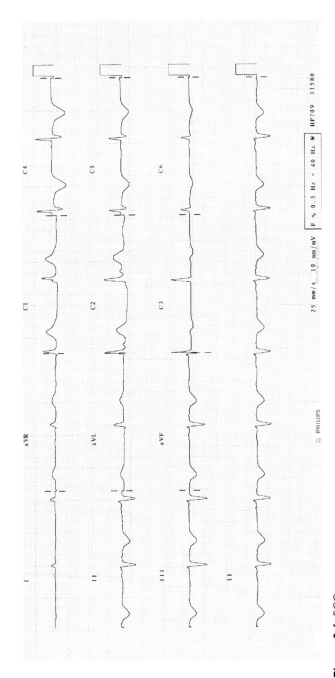

Figure 3.6 ECG

55. **A 76-year-old man presented in clinic complaining of worsening breathlessness. He had a history of hypertension, hypercholesterolaemia, paroxysmal atrial fibrillation, trans-ischaemic attack, gout, and arthritis. On examination, his pulse was irregular at 90 bpm and his blood pressure was 147/90 mmHg. He had no murmurs and his chest was clear to auscultation. His regular medication included ibuprofen 200 mg tds, bisoprolol 2.5 mg od, ramipril 5 mg od, allopurinol 400 mg od, simvastatin 20 mg and bendroflumethizide 2.5 mg od. What change to his medication is most important to reduce his cardiovascular risk?**

   A. Add aspirin 75 mg od
   B. Add furosemide 40 mg od
   C. Add warfarin
   D. Increase bisoprolol to 5 mg od
   E. Increase ramipril to 7.5 mg od

56. **A 23-year-old man is admitted to the emergency department after taking a line of cocaine and an amphetamine tablet at a party. He started feeling faint, and on admission his BP is 110/50 and his ventricular rate is 150. His ECG is consistent with a paroxysmal atrial tachycardia. Which of the following is the most appropriate initial therapy for him?**

   A. Carotid sinus massage
   B. Verapamil
   C. Diltiazem
   D. Amiodarone
   E. Flecanide

57. **The following abnormalities cause a reversed split second heart sound, except:**

   A. Pulmonary stenosis
   B. Patent ductus arteriosus
   C. Left bundle branch block
   D. Aortic stenosis
   E. Right ventricular pacing

58. **A 45-year-old man is admitted with chest pain relieved by bending forwards. On examination he has a soft rub audible at the left lower sternal edge but no signs of tamponade. His ECG shows sinus rhythm with widespread ST elevation of up to 1 mm. Echocardiography reveals a small pericardial effusion without evidence of tamponade. He was started on prednisolone for acute pericarditis. What is the best description of steroid treatment in this condition?**

    A. It is usually used as an adjunct for colchicine therapy
    B. It is usually used as an adjunct for NSAID therapy
    C. It has similar efficacy whether administered intrapericardially or systemically
    D. It reduces the risk of disease recurrence
    E. It should be administered at high doses for at least one month before slow tapering

59. **An 87-year-old woman with Alzheimer's dementia presents from her nursing home due to concern from her carers regarding her mobility. On further questioning it is established that over the last two days she has spent increasing time in her bed, has become more confused than usual, and has been expectorating purulent sputum. She has not complained of any chest pains. Admission observations are as follows: oxygen saturations of 84% on room air, respiratory rate of 24 breaths per minute, pulse of 160 bpm, blood pressure of 90/30 mmHg and temperature of 38.0°C. Clinical examination reveals coarse crepitations at the left base and an irregularly irregular pulse of 160 bpm. Chest radiograph confirms left basal consolidation. An electrocardiogram confirms atrial fibrillation with fast ventricular response (rate 160 bpm) with marked ST segment depression in the lateral chest leads. Your house officer contacts you regarding this patient because he is concerned about one of her blood results from the initial battery of tests sent in the accident and emergency department. The troponin T is elevated at 730 ng/l (upper limit of normal = 14 ng/l). Other bloods include: WCC 20, CRP 250, urea 3, creatinine 57. In which classification of myocardial infarction (MI) does this woman's clinical scenario place her?**

    A. Type 1 MI
    B. Type 2 MI
    C. Type 3 MI
    D. Type 4a MI
    E. Type 5 MI

60. **A 34-year-old man is found to have hypertrophic cardiomyopathy. As part of his risk assessment he underwent a series of investigations including echocardiography, exercise tolerance testing, and Holter monitoring. Which of the following are regarded as major risk factors for sudden cardiac death?**

A. Dynamic left ventricular outflow tract gradient obstruction
B. Frequent ventricular ectopic beats on Holter monitoring
C. No change in blood pressure during exercise tolerance testing
D. Paroxysmal atrial fibrillation on Holter monitoring
E. Septal wall thickness of 20 mm

61. **Oral and sublingual nitrates are important cardiovascular drugs. Which of the following best describes their use in clinical practice?**

A. They are contraindicated in constrictive pericarditis
B. They are recommended in the treatment of angina associated with hypertrophic cardiomyopathy
C. They reduce the production of nitric oxide
D. They should be avoided in anterior myocardial infarction
E. They should not be given to patients with glaucoma

62. **A 56-year-old man was referred for genetic screening following a diagnosis of hypertrophic cardiomyopathy. The commonest genetic cause of sarcomeric hypertrophic cardiomyopathy is due to mutations in the gene encoding for which one of the following proteins?**

A. Alpha tropomyosin
B. Beta myosin heavy chain
C. Cardiac troponin T
D. Essential light chain of myosin
E. Titin

63. **An 18-year-old man was referred to the cardiology clinic because of the finding of a loud systolic murmur at an insurance medical examination. He reported that this had been present since infancy but he had been a healthy child with normal milestones. On examination he had a loud systolic murmur but no other abnormality. What is the most likely diagnosis?**

A. Atrial septal defect
B. Congenital aortic stenosis
C. Congenital pulmonary atresia
D. Fallot's tetralogy
E. Ventricular septal defect

64. **A patient presents with hypertension, acute pulmonary oedema with known poor LV function, and no valvular heart disease. The most appropriate immediate management option is:**
    A. Dobutamine
    B. Intra-aortic balloon pumping
    C. Intravenous nitrates
    D. Oral beta blockers
    E. Intravenous furosemide

65. **A 27-year-old woman presents to you with exertional chest pain, breathlessness, and episodes of collapse. She has a family history of her father dying of ischaemic heart disease in his fifties. Routine blood tests are normal, her blood pressure is 110/70, her total cholesterol is 5.8, and her ECG is as shown in Figure 3.7. What is the most likely diagnosis?**
    A. Angina
    B. Atypical chest pain and incidental right bundle branch block
    C. Brugada syndrome
    D. Congenital long QT syndrome, type I
    E. Primary pulmonary hypertension

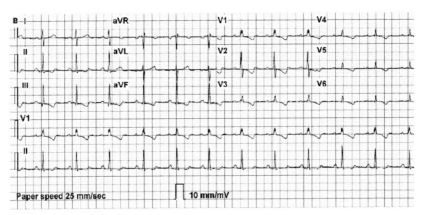

Figure 3.7 ECG at presentation

66. **A six-month-old boy is brought to casualty having had a sudden episode of breathlessness. He is clubbed and mildly cyanosed. There is a horizontal scar parasternally in the right second intercostal space and a harsh ejection murmur at the base of the heart. What is the most likely underlying diagnosis?**
    A. Atrial septal defect with Eisenmenger's syndrome
    B. Congenitally corrected transposition of the great arteries
    C. Fallot's tetralogy
    D. Hypoplastic left heart syndrome
    E. Ventricular septal defect with Eisenmenger's syndrome

67. **A 35-year-old woman presents with increasing shortness of breath. On examination the lungs are clear. The pulse is 80 bpm and regular. The blood pressure is 130/60 mmHg. Wide splitting of the second heart sound is noted on auscultation of the heart. Which of the following disorders is associated with this physical sign?**

    A. Aortic stenosis
    B. Patent ductus arteriosus
    C. Atrial septal defect (ASD)
    D. Pulmonary embolism
    E. Left bundle branch block

68. **A 32-year-old man presents with retrosternal chest ache which is worse on lying flat and better on leaning forward. He says this began 24 hours earlier and is worse on deep breathing. There is mild shortness of breath, and he has had a cold over the past week or so. Examination reveals a BP of 135/72 and a pulse of 80. His ECG reveals widespread saddle-shaped ST elevation. Troponin is elevated at 2.1. Which of the following is the most appropriate treatment?**

    A. Diclofenac
    B. Aspirin
    C. Low molecular weight heparin
    D. Angioplasty
    E. Thrombolysis

69. **A 69-year-old man comes to the clinic for review of his cardiac failure. He has increasing shortness of breath and his family have had to move his bed downstairs. On examination he is short of breath at rest, his BP is 105/81, and his pulse is 83. He has bilateral crackles on auscultation of his chest and bilateral pitting oedema of both ankles. Medication includes ramipril 10 mg, furosemide 80 mg, spironolactone 25 mg, and carvedilol 12.5 mg BD. ECG reveals left bundle branch block which has been present since a myocardial infarction some six years earlier. Which of the following is the most appropriate next step?**

    A. Increase his spironolactone
    B. Increase his carvedilol
    C. Add digoxin
    D. Add metolazone
    E. Refer for cardiac resynchronization therapy

70. **A 62-year-old man comes to the clinic for review of his heart failure. He tells you that he has increasing shortness of breath and has to sleep in a chair sitting up for most of the week and can't make it up the stairs. Medication includes ramipril 10 mg and furosemide 80 mg. His BP is 135/82. Investigations: Haemoglobin 12.1 g/dl (13.5–17.7), white cells 5.4 x 10⁹/l (4–11), platelets 230 x 10⁹/l (150–400), sodium 138 mmol/l (135–146), potassium 4.5 mmol/l (3.5–5), creatinine 135 micromol/l (79–118), ejection fraction 28%. Which of the following is the most appropriate next intervention?**

    A. Add bisoprolol 2.5 mg
    B. Increase furosemide to 120 mg
    C. Add candesartan 4 mg
    D. Add spironolactone 100 mg
    E. Add digoxin 125 mcg

71. **A 62-year-old man with a history of hypertension is admitted after a road traffic accident. He rear shunted another car, and on initial admission to the emergency department he is complaining of chest pain from a steering wheel blow to the chest. Medication includes ramipril, amlodipine, and atorvastatin, although he has never suffered a previous infarct. On examination his BP is 165/100, his pulse is 86 and regular. There is a seat belt and steering wheel bruise to his anterior chest. You are asked to review him three hours later on the observation ward because of continued chest pain. Investigations: Haemoglobin 12.9 g/dl (13.5–17.7), white cells 8.3 x10⁹/l (4–11), platelets 234 x10⁹/l (150–400), sodium 141 mmol/l (135–146), potassium 5.1 mmol/l (3.5–5), creatinine 132 micromol/l (79–118), ECG—T wave inversion, troponin 0.6. Which of the following is the most appropriate intervention?**

    A. Simple analgesia
    B. Low molecular weight heparin
    C. Angiography
    D. Aspirin
    E. Aspirin and clopidogrel

72. **A 79-year-old man is reviewed in the cardiology clinic after suffering a collapse while shopping in the local supermarket. He has been suffering from increasing angina over the preceding three months for which he had been prescribed atenolol 50 mg od and isosorbide mononitrate 20 mg bd. On examination he has a regular pulse of 70 bpm, a blood pressure of 125/100 mmHg, and an ejection systolic murmur. Echocardiography reveals aortic stenosis with a peak gradient measured by Doppler of 65 mmHg. What is the most appropriate next step in his management?**
    A. Aortic valve replacement
    B. Aortic valvotomy
    C. Increase atenolol dose
    D. Reduce isosorbide mononitrate dose
    E. Start amlodipine 5 mg od

73. **A 39-year-old man is reviewed in clinic complaining of increasing shortness of breath, exertional chest pain, decreased exercise tolerance, and pre-syncope. He was diagnosed with hypertrophic cardiomyopathy following his brother's sudden death two years earlier. On examination his blood pressure is 150/90 mmHg, he has a double apex beat and an ejection systolic murmur. Investigations: chest X-ray: cardiomegaly and interstitial pulmonary oedema; echocardiography: marked septal hypertrophy and a left ventricular outflow tract gradient of 75 mmHg. Which of the following is the most appropriate next treatment?**
    A. Oral furosemide
    B. Oral spironolactone
    C. Oral valsartan
    D. Implantable cardioverter defibrillator
    E. Surgical myomectomy

74. **A 67-year-old man presents with reduced exercise intolerance and progressive peripheral oedema. Which of the following features is most useful to distinguish pericardial constriction from restrictive cardiomyopathy?**
    A. Calcification on chest X-ray
    B. Equalization of left and right ventricular diastolic pressures at cardiac catheterization
    C. Low voltages on ECG
    D. Presence of Kussmaul's sign
    E. Tissue Doppler abnormalities on echocardiography

75. **A 59-year-old man is admitted with shortness of breath and ankle swelling. He complains of 'arthritis' in both knees recently, for which he has been taking NSAIDs. He denies any chest pain. On examination, he is in sinus rhythm with a blood pressure of 110/70 mmHg. Jugular venous pressure is elevated 4 cm and he has sacral oedema. In his chest he has bilateral basal crepitations. There is mild hepatomegaly, but no ascites and small testes. He has bilateral knee effusions. What is the cause of his present condition**

    A. Amyloidosis
    B. Haemochromatosis
    C. Hypopituitarism
    D. Klinefelter's syndrome
    E. Sarcoidosis

76. **A 32-year-old injecting drug user presents with rigors and a fever of 39.4°C. Admission observations reveal a regular pulse of 100 bpm and a blood pressure of 120/65 mmHg. Inspection reveals giant 'v' waves visible in the jugular venous pulse and auscultation reveals a pan-systolic murmur audible maximally at the lower left sternal edge. Which is the most likely cardiac lesion that explains this clinical picture?**

    A. Mitral regurgitation
    B. Coarctation of the aorta
    C. Ventricular septal defect
    D. Tricuspid regurgitation
    E. Aortic stenosis

77. **The cardiovascular effects of neuromuscular disorders are important determinants of morbidity and mortality. Which of these conditions is most commonly associated with dilated cardiomyopathy?**

    A. Duchenne muscular dystrophy
    B. Inclusion body myositis
    C. Limb girdle muscular dystrophy
    D. Myasthenia gravis
    E. Myotonic dystrophy

78. **A 29-year-old athlete comes to the emergency room for review. He has been suffering pleuritic chest pains and symptoms of a cold over the past few days and has been unable to train due to shortness of breath. On examination he has a mild fever of 37.8°C, a BP of 110/62, and a pulse of 82. His ECG reveals saddle-shaped ST elevation and his troponin is raised at 2.1. Which of the following is the most likely diagnosis?**

    A. Viral pericarditis
    B. Viral myocarditis
    C. NSTEMI
    D. STEMI
    E. Subacute bacterial endocarditis

79. **An 80-year-old woman presents with fevers and rigors. She is febrile at 39°C. Examination reveals splinter haemorrhages and a new pan-systolic murmur heard maximally at the apex. Three sets of blood cultures are taken from separate sites and trans-oesophageal echocardiography (TOE) confirms evidence of a vegetation on the mitral valve, suggestive of a diagnosis of endocarditis, but limited valvular compromise. The blood cultures subsequently grow Streptococcus bovis and appropriate antibiotics are commenced. The patient responds well to antibiotic therapy and is subsequently discharged. What is the most appropriate next management step?**

    A. Repeat trans-oesophageal echocardiography (TOE)
    B. Trans-thoracic echocardiography (TTE)
    C. Cardiac magnetic resonance imaging (MRI) scan
    D. Referral for consideration of colonoscopy
    E. Referral to cardiothoracic surgeons

80. **A 35-year-old man is admitted on the medical take with palpitations, but is otherwise well. His ECG shows a regular narrow complex tachycardia with a rate of 140 bpm. There is no evidence of bundle branch block or delta waves. The blood pressure is 125/75 and there are no signs of shock, myocardial ischaemia, or heart failure. You try vagal manoeuvres which are not successful in cardioverting him. Which medication should you try next?**

    A. Adrenaline
    B. Amiodarone
    C. Adenosine
    D. Digoxin
    E. None of the above—go straight for DC cardioversion

81. **A 26-year-old woman who has a previous history of paroxysmal SVT presents with palpitations. These have lasted for around 30 minutes and she has not been able to resolve them herself using the Valsalva manoeuvre. She is eight months pregnant. On examination her BP is 105/60, and her ventricular rate is around 185 bpm on the monitor. Her chest is clear and she is apyrexial. A 12-lead ECG reveals a narrow complex tachycardia. Investigations: Hb 12.1, WCC 7.2, PLT 201, Na 137, K 4.1, Cr 88. Which of the following is the most appropriate therapy for her?**

    A. Amiodarone
    B. Verapamil
    C. Propranolol
    D. Adenosine
    E. Propafenone

82. **A 32-year-old woman is referred for review because of palpitations. She has no other past medical history and is taking no regular medication. On examination she has a regular pulse of 64 bpm, a normal venous pressure, and a blood pressure of 128/74 mmHg. She has fixed splitting of the second heart sound and a systolic murmur. What is the most likely underlying condition?**

    A. Atrial septal defect
    B. Left bundle branch block
    C. Pulmonary atresia
    D. Pulmonary stenosis
    E. Ventricular septal defect

83. **A 35-year-old man is brought to the emergency room by ambulance after collapsing in his bedroom in the early hours of the morning. According to his wife he woke in the early hours, his chest sounded bubbly, and he was incredibly short of breath. He has a past history of lens dislocation, left shoulder and right patellar dislocation. On examination his BP is 105/60 (equal in both arms), his pulse is 94 and regular. He is in pulmonary oedema on auscultation of the chest. There is an early diastolic murmur over the aortic area. Which of the following diagnoses fits best with the history and examination?**

    A. Mitral regurgitation
    B. Myocarditis
    C. Aortic regurgitation
    D. Aortic dissection
    E. Aortitis

84. A 43-year-old man is admitted with a two-week history of cough, dyspnoea, and sweating. He has no significant past medical history but is known to keep pigeons. On examination he has a temperature of 38.2°C, a regular pulse of 80 bpm, and a blood pressure of 125/65 mmHg. He has a systolic murmur. Investigations: Full blood count: Hb 10.9, WCC 12.3, PLT 203; Biochemistry: Na 137, K 4.3, Cr 102; Chest X-ray: left lower lobe consolidation; Blood cultures: no growth in three sets; Echocardiography: moderate mitral regurgitation with valve vegetations. Which of the following is the most likely causative organism?

    A. *C. psittaci*
    B. *S. aureus*
    C. *S. epidermidis*
    D. *S. pneumoniae*
    E. *S. viridans*

85. A 78-year-old man with a background of chronic hypertension, asthma, and recurrent stroke disease is admitted to your ward overnight. You are asked to review the patient because the nurses are concerned that his heart rate is around 150 bpm. On arrival at the bedside the patient is alert and converses with you appropriately. He has no chest pain. Clinically, there is no evidence of heart failure. Blood pressure is 130/90 mmHg. He has bilateral audible carotid bruits. A glance at his drug card shows his regular medications to be aspirin, dipyridamole, lisinopril, and simvastatin. An urgent ECG reveals a regular, narrow complex tachycardia (rate 150 bpm) consistent with an SVT. Vagal manoeuvres are attempted but there is no change in the patient's underlying rhythm or rate. Which of the following is the most appropriate intervention to undertake?

    A. Carotid sinus massage
    B. IV adenosine
    C. IV metoprolol
    D. Immediate synchronized DC cardioversion
    E. IV diltiazem

86. A 33-year-old man is admitted with fever, sweating, and cough with dry phlegm. He has abused heroin for several years and has just started methadone. Investigations show: Haemoglobin 11.8 mg/l, white cell count 17.3 x 10⁹/l, urea 12.8 mmol/l, serum creatinine 187 micromol/l. Chest X-ray—small right pleural effusion and several nodular densities, one of which is cavitating. Urinalysis blood 2+. What is the likely cause of his illness?

    A. Acute HIV infection
    B. Goodpasture's syndrome
    C. Henoch–Schonlein purpura
    D. Infective endocarditis
    E. Wegener's granulomatosis

87. **A 62-year-old woman presents to the clinic with progressively increasing shortness of breath on minimal exertion. She has a past history of rheumatic fever as a teenager and was admitted two months earlier with pulmonary oedema. On examination, she has a malar flush, her pulse is regular at 85 bpm, and her blood pressure is 135/92 mmHg. She has a loud first heart sound and a mid-diastolic murmur. Investigations: Echocardiography: severe mitral stenosis with significant mitral valve calcification. What is the most appropriate management?**

    A. Bisoprolol 1.25 mg od
    B. Closed valvotomy
    C. Mitral valve replacement
    D. Percutaneous balloon valvotomy
    E. Ramipril 2.5 mg od

88. **A 39-year-old woman is admitted to the emergency department with palpitations. She has had multiple episodes of shortness of breath and rapid irregular palpitations on a number of occasions over the past 6–9 months. On examination, she has reverted to sinus rhythm, with a BP of 132/72 and a pulse of 75 regular. She has a mid-diastolic murmur and bilateral ankle swelling. Which of the following is true of the condition?**

    A. Nitrates may relieve breathlessness
    B. ACE inhibitors are contraindicated
    C. Furosemide is contraindicated because it reduces pre-load
    D. ECHO and Doppler are inaccurate in determining the degree of stenosis
    E. Anticoagulation is only recommended if there is thrombus in the left atrium

89. **A 54-year-old woman was admitted to the A&E department following a collapse. Shortly after arrival she was observed to lose consciousness for a few seconds during which her ECG monitor showed polymorphic ventricular tachycardia. She has a past medical history of hypertension and was being treated for a chest infection. She reported taking magnesium dietary supplements. Her father and grandfather had both died suddenly in their thirties but the cause was unknown. Which of the patient's medications is most likely to have contributed to her collapse?**

    A. Aspirin
    B. Atenolol
    C. Erythromycin
    D. Magnesium glycerophosphate
    E. Spironolactone

90. **A 67-year-old woman attends the emergency department because of palpitations lasting 40 minutes. She has a history of previous anterior myocardial infarction. Her medication includes aspirin 75 mg od, simvastatin 40 mg nocte, ramipril 5 mg od, and bisoprolol 5 mg od. On examination she has an irregular pulse of 130 bpm and a blood pressure of 120/60 mmHg. On auscultation of her chest she has bilateral basal crackles. Investigations: Full blood count: Hb 12.3, WCC 7.8, Plt 192; Electrolytes: Na 138, K 4.1, Cr 122; ECG: atrial fibrillation with an average ventricular rate of 130 bpm, Q waves in leads V1 to V4, ST segment depression in leads V4–V6. Which of the following is the most appropriate initial intravenous medication?**

    A. Amiodarone
    B. Digoxin
    C. Flecainide
    D. Metoprolol
    E. Verapamil

91. **An 86-year-old woman is admitted with unstable angina. Over the course of her admission she develops increasing shortness of breath. An urgent chest X-ray is performed. Which of the following is least consistent with a diagnosis of heart failure?**

    A. A unilateral right-sided pleural effusion
    B. Enlarged cardiac silhouette
    C. Prominent lower zone vasculature versus upper zone
    D. Horizontal lines in the periphery of the lung bases
    E. Multiple small, ill-defined air space opacities

92. **A 52-year-old man comes to the clinic complaining of chest pain which can come on at any time of day, including whilst exercising or after a meal, or even whilst sitting down. He says it is relieved by belching. He smokes 20 cigarettes per day, has impaired glucose tolerance, and is treated for hypertension with ramipril 10 mg. On examination in the clinic his BMI is 31, his BP is 155/81, and his pulse is 78 and regular. Heart sounds are normal and there are no signs of cardiac failure. His resting ECG, U&E, and FBC are normal. Which of the following is the most appropriate investigation for his angina?**

    A. Exercise test
    B. MIBI scan
    C. Echocardiogram
    D. MR angiography
    E. Traditional angiography

93. **A 34-year-old city trader is admitted from a Christmas party after collapsing with central crushing chest pain. He admits to being a habitual cocaine user, having used two lines during the course of the evening. He also smokes 40 cigarettes per day. On examination he is pale, sweaty, and in pain. His BP is 165/100, pulse is 90 and regular. He has bilateral crackles on auscultation of the chest. ECG reveals evidence of anterior ST elevation. On arrival he is given GTN, oxygen, and aspirin. Which of the following treatments is recommended next?**

    A. Atenolol
    B. Angiography
    C. Bisoprolol
    D. TPA
    E. Verapamil

94. **A 61-year-old man is recovering on the cardiology ward some three days after an inferior myocardial infarction when he suddenly becomes acutely short of breath. By the time the nurses ask you to see him he is in left ventricular failure with a BP of 130/80, a pulse of 100, and a quiet systolic murmur. Which of the following is the most appropriate initial treatment?**

    A. Furosemide
    B. Diamorphine
    C. NIPPV
    D. Nitroprusside
    E. Dobutamine

95. **A 74-year-old man presents with worsening shortness of breath and a marked decrease in his exercise tolerance. He had an anterior MI four years earlier and has been troubled by symptoms of heart failure since then. On examination his blood pressure is 135/75 mmHg, his pulse is 80 and regular, and he has signs of biventricular heart failure. His medications include aspirin, diltiazem, lisinopril, furosemide, isosorbide mononitrate, diltiazem, and simvastatin. Investigations: Hb 12.9 g/dl, WCC 6.4 x 10^9/l, PLT 208 x 10^9/l, Na 137 mmol/l, K 4.3 mmol/l, Cr 141 micromol/l. ECG: Anterior Q waves. CXR: Cardiomegaly, interstitial oedema. What is the most appropriate medication change to improve his prognosis?**

    A. Bumetanide in place of furosemide
    B. Carvedilol in place of atenolol
    C. Digoxin in addition to current therapy
    D. Valsartan in place of lisinopril
    E. Verapamil in place of diltiazem

96. **A 54-year-old man is admitted to the emergency room with central crushing chest pain which began in the early hours of the morning and was accompanied by severe nausea and sweating. He smokes 20 cigarettes per day and is obese, with impaired glucose tolerance. On examination he has a regular pulse of 82 bpm and a blood pressure of 145/82 mmHg. His ECG showed anterior ST elevation which resolved over 30 minutes with the use of GTN. His troponin T at 12 h was less than 12 ng/l. What is the most likely diagnosis?**

    A. Coronary artery vasospasm
    B. Non-ST elevation myocardial infarction
    C. Pericarditis
    D. ST elevation myocardial infarction
    E. Unstable angina

97. **A 46-year-old type I diabetic with peripheral vascular disease attends complaining of severe abdominal pain 20–60 minutes after food for one month. He does not drink alcohol and gave up smoking some five years previously. As a result of his pain, he was afraid to eat and had lost 10 kg in weight. He has undergone gastroscopy, small bowel meal, and CT scan of his abdomen which were normal, as also were his liver function tests, apart from an albumin of 32 g/l. His urea was 12.2 mmol/l and serum creatinine 156 micromol/l. Serum amylase was normal. What is the cause of his abdominal pain?**

    A. Autonomic gastroparesis
    B. Chronic pancreatitis
    C. Mesenteric angina
    D. Non-organic pain
    E. Porphyria

98. **A 33-year-old man who has been previously investigated for recurrent shoulder dislocation comes to the emergency room. He collapsed in the supermarket complaining of excrutiating pain going from the front of his chest to between his shoulder blades. His BP is elevated at 155/95, there are bilateral basal crackles consistent with pulmonary oedema, and a murmur consistent with aortic regurgitation. ECG reveals inferior ST elevation. Which of the following is the most appropriate next step?**

    A. Chest X-ray
    B. Thrombolysis
    C. Angioplasty and stenting
    D. Troponin
    E. CKMB

99. A 52-year-old man is admitted with a 36-hour history of increasingly severe headache and nausea. He is normally well and has not consulted the doctor in the past three years. On examination in the emergency room he has a blood pressure of 180/115, and retinal changes consistent with grade 3 hypertensive retinopathy. He is not in pulmonary oedema and his pulse is 85 and regular. A CT head is unremarkable. His creatinine is mildly elevated at 135 micromol/l. Which of the following is the most appropriate target for diastolic blood pressure lowering in the first 24 hours?

    A. 110 mmHg
    B. 100 mmHg
    C. 90 mmHg
    D. 85 mmHg
    E. 80 mmHg

100. You review a 69-year-old man with chronic renal failure in the clinic. You are thinking about management of his blood pressure. Which of the following is likely to provide the best estimate of his blood pressure control?

    A. Pre-dialysis BP
    B. Post-dialysis BP
    C. Inter-dialysis BP
    D. Inter-dialysis ABPM
    E. During dialysis BP

101. A 62-year-old man is reviewed in the cardiology clinic. He has a history of ischaemic heart disease, type 2 diabetes, and heart failure. He says he has been started on some new medication since his last appointment and is complaining of severe, painful, mouth ulceration. Which of the following medications is most likely to be the cause?

    A. Amlodipine
    B. Gliclazide
    C. Metformin
    D. Nicorandil
    E. Ramipril

102. A 62-year-old man suffers a cardiac arrest and dies in the hospital car park. He had a long history of type 2 diabetes and hypertension, and smoked 20 cigarettes per day. According to his wife he had sudden onset central crushing chest pain radiating to both arms. Which of the following is the most likely cause of death?

    A. Ruptured ventricular septal defect
    B. Acute mitral regurgitation
    C. Thoracic aorta dissection
    D. Ventricular fibrillation
    E. Ruptured left ventricle

103. **A 40 year old Afro-Caribbean woman comes to the clinic for review. She has hypertension and has failed to tolerate amlodipine 5 mg daily due to ankle swelling. Her BP is still elevated at 155/98. Which of the following is the intervention of choice?**
    A. Bendroflumethiazide
    B. Hydrochlorthiazide
    C. Ramipril
    D. Valsartan
    E. Indapamide

104. **A 44-year-old man presents to the emergency department with central crushing chest pain radiating to his left arm after a night out with friends. He admits to extensive use of cocaine, alcohol, and says he smokes 20–40 cigarettes/day. On examination his BP is 182/95, pulse is 100 and regular. His heart sounds are normal and there are bilateral crackles on auscultation of his chest. ECG reveals anterolateral ST depression. He is given IV morphine but is still in pain. Which of the following medications is most likely to be effective in managing his chest pain?**
    A. Bisoprolol
    B. Glyceryl trinitrate
    C. Diazepam
    D. Fondaparinux
    E. Clopidogrel

105. **When considering myocardial infarction as a consequence of percutaneous coronary intervention (PCI), which of the following is true?**
    A. Periprocedural myocardial infarction occurs in less than 5% of cases of PCI
    B. A periprocedural myocardial infarction is defined as that which gives a rise in troponin T or troponin I at least three times the upper limit of normal 8–12 hours after the procedure
    C. All patients undergoing PCI should be screened for periprocedural myocardial infarction after the procedure
    D. Periprocedural myocardial infarction is a marker of atherosclerotic burden rather than an indicator of patient prognosis
    E. Younger patients are at greater risk of periprocedural myocardial infarction

106. **A 62 year-old woman presents with cardiac-sounding central chest pain. She has a history of type 2 diabetes mellitus for which she takes metformin monotherapy. She has had previous percutaneous coronary intervention to her mid-left anterior descending artery with deployment of a drug-eluting stent over fuve years ago. On examination her BP is 155/90, pulse is 92 and regular. Which of the following is the most likely diagnosis?**

    A. Left anterior descending in-stent restenosis
    B. Left anterior descending stent thrombosis
    C. Left circumflex artery disease
    D. Right coronary artery disease
    E. Left anterior descending coronary artery spasm

107. **A 62-year-old man is reviewed in the heart failure clinic. He is able to walk only a few yards before getting short of breath and has to sleep downstairs. His medical history includes COPD for which he took salbutamol, tiotropium, and high-dose seretide. On examination his pulse is regular at 64 bpm and his blood pressure is 105/70 mmHg. There were bilateral crackles on auscultation of his chest and mild ankle oedema. His medication includes ramipril 10 mg, bumetanide 3 mg, bisoprolol 10 mg, spironolactone 25 mg and digoxin 62.5 mcg. Investigations: Hb 11.9 g/dl, WCC 7.6 x10(9)/L, PLT 240 x10(9)/L, Na+ 132 mmol/L, K+ 5.0 mmol/L, creatinine 129 µmol/L, FEV1 40% of predicted. He has asked about the possibility of heart transplant. Which of the following would be the most significant contraindication?**

    A. Age
    B. COPD with decreased FEV1
    C. Heart failure NYHA class III
    D. Hypotension
    E. Renal impairment

108. **A 62-year-old man with biventricular failure who is treated with aspirin, atorvastatin, ramipril, bisoprolol, and spironolactone comes to the clinic for review. His heart failure symptoms are stable, as are his full blood count and urea and electrolytes. His main complaint at this appointment is of gynaecomastia. Which of the following is the most appropriate course of action?**

    A. Stop his spironolactone
    B. Switch his spironolactone for eplerenone
    C. Switch his spironolactone for valsartan
    D. Switch his spironolactone for furosemide
    E. Stop his ramipril

109. A 56-year-old man was admitted with acute anterior myocardial infarction. He initially recovered well but 36 hours later collapsed on the ward. On examination his BP was 85/50mmHg, his pulse was 100 bpm and regular. He was peripherally shut down, and there was a loud systolic murmur. He was in peripheral oedema with a respiratory rate of 30 bpm. What is the most likely cause of his sudden deterioration?

    A. Aortic dissection
    B. Atrial septal defect
    C. Mitral valve rupture
    D. Ventricular free wall rupture
    E. Ventricular septal defect

110. A 62-year-old woman was referred to the cardiology clinic. She described increasing shortness of breath despite maximum tolerated ACE inhibitior dose and was able to walk only 50–60 m before needing to stop. Her past included an anterior myocardial infarction three years previously, and she continued to smoke five cigarettes per day. On examination she had a regular pulse at 80 bpm and a BP of 110/70 mmHg. She had no murmur but there were bibasal crackles on auscultation of her chest. She did not have ankle swelling. Investigations: Hb 11.0 g/dl, WCC 7.1 × 10(9)/L, PLT 181 × 10(9)/L, Na+ 137 mmol/L, K+ 4.6 mmol/L, Creatinine 131 µmol/L. ECG: sinus rhythm 80 beats-per-minute, left bundle branch block. Echocardiography: Anterior hypokinesia, left ventricular ejection fraction 30%. Which of the following is the most appropriate intervention?

    A. Cardiac resynchronization therapy
    B. Furosemide
    C. Indapamide
    D. Bisoprolol
    E. Valsartan

111. A 62-year-old man with chronic stable angina and heart failure comes to the clinic for review. Current medication includes aspirin, atorvastatin, ramipril, bisoprolol, spironolactone, and furosemide. His exercise tolerance is currently limited by angina to approximately 100 yards on the flat or one flight of stairs. On examination his BP is 132/82, pulse is 90. He is not in fluid overload and his most recent creatinine is 115. Which of the following medications is most likely to impact on his prognosis?

    A. Amlodipine
    B. Nicorandil
    C. Diltiazem
    D. Ivabradine
    E. Isosorbide dinitrate

112. A 64-year-old man presents to the emergency department with central chest pain radiating down his left arm, lasting for 90 minutes, which began whilst he was mowing his lawn. He smokes 20 cigarettes per day and takes amlodipine for management of his blood pressure. On examination his BP is 155/90, pulse is 95 and regular. He is pain free at rest, having been given 2.5mg of diamorphine IV by the paramedic crew. He has no murmurs, and there is no evidence of left ventricular failure. He is given 300 mg of aspirin and 300 mg of clopidogrel. Investigations: Hb 13.9, WCC 8.9, PLT 209, Na 138, K 4.7, Cr 108, Troponin 0.9 (5hrs), ECG inferior ST depression. Which of the following is the most appropriate next step?

    A. Abciximab
    B. Fraxiparin
    C. Enoxiparin
    D. Unfractionated heparin
    E. Fondaparinux

113. A 68-year-old man with a history of three previous myocardial infarctions and biventricular heart failure attends the clinic for review. His heart failure appears stable, although he has suffered twice weekly attacks of angina over the past four months. His medication includes ramipril, bisoprolol, furosemide, aspirin, and atorvastatin. On examination his BP is 135/72 mmHg and his pulse is 85 bpm and regular. What is the most appropriate additional medication?

    A. Amlodipine
    B. Diltiazem
    C. Isosorbide dinitrate
    D. Ivabradine
    E. Nebivolol

114. A 72-year-old woman presents with a tachyarrhythmia. She collapsed during a service at the local church some 30 minutes earlier. On arrival in the emergency department her BP is 100/60, pulse is 160 and regular. ECG reveals a ventricular rate of 160 and a right bundle branch block like pattern. Which of the following features would favour VT rather than SVT?

    A. Triphasic QRS in V6
    B. Monophasic R in V1
    C. R to S ratio>1 in V6
    D. Heart rate 160
    E. Systolic BP of 100

115. **A 74-year-old woman comes to the emergency department with rapidly worsening shortness of breath and palpitations. She suffered a previous inferior infarct some four years ago and is currently treated with ramipril, bumetanide, aspirin, and atorvastatin. Her BP is 105/70, pulse is 125 (atrial fibrillation). There are crackles to the mid zones bilaterally, and pitting oedema to the mid shins. Her creatinine is 132 micromol/l and her potassium is 3.9 mmol/l. Which of the following is the most appropriate intervention?**

    A. Bisoprolol
    B. Digoxin
    C. Amiodarone
    D. Flecanide
    E. Diltiazem

116. **A 70-year-old woman is admitted to the emergency department with acute shortness of breath. She suffered an inferior myocardial infarction three months ago and was discharged taking bisoprolol, ramipril, furosemide, atorvastatin, and aspirin. She has not been taking her medication over the preceding five days as she has been travelling on the bus to look after her grandchildren. On examination she has a regular pulse of 95 bpm and a blood pressure of 168/88 mmHg. She has extensive crackles on auscultation consistent with heart failure. Her oxygen saturation on 8 L/min oxygen is 92%. Following intravenous GTN and furosemide she remains distressed with a respiratory rate of 30 breaths per minute. Her blood pressure is 133/78 mmHg and her oxygen saturation is 94%. What is the most appropriate next step in her management?**

    A. Intravenous diamorphine
    B. Intravenous dobutamine
    C. Intravenous dopamine
    D. Intubation and ventilation
    E. Non-invasive ventilation

CARDIOLOGY

3

ANSWERS

1. A. Staphylococcus aureus

Staphylococcus aureus alone accounts for 50–70% of cases of endocarditis in IV drug abusers. Large vegetations are typical. Abscesses in the fibro-cardiac skeleton tissue or the myocardium are much more likely to be found in acute bacterial endocarditis than subacute bacterial endocarditis. All listed organisms are capable of causing this type of infection so obtaining blood cultures is the cornerstone in the management of such cases. The test result would help guide the appropriate use of sensitive antibiotics.

Fernández Guerrero ML et al., Endocarditis caused by Staphylococcus aureus: a reappraisal of the epidemiologic, clinical, and pathologic manifestations with analysis of factors determining outcome. *Medicine* (Baltimore) 2009;88:122.

2. C. Long diastolic murmur

A long murmur is actually a sign of mild aortic regurgitation, because in severe AR, the ventricular pressure rises rapidly during diastole due to the large regurgitant volume. This in turn rapidly reduces the pressure gradient between the aorta and the ventricle; thus flow rapidly slows and the murmur is lost in mid diastole. This clinical sign is the clinical correlate of the short pressure half time of the slope of the AR Doppler trace that is obtained during echo assessment.

Ali Khavandi , Essential Revision Notes for the Cardiology KBA, Oxford University Press, 2014, chapter 5, Valvular heart disease.

3. C. Reassure her

This patient has no sinister features consistent with her palpitations. Features that suggest a sinister cause for premature ventricular ectopics include: occurring frequently (6 or more beats/min); PVE in bigeminal rhythm; PVE in short runs of ventricular tachycardia; PVE exhibiting R-on-T phenomenon; PVE associated with serious organic heart disease and left ventricular decompensation. Therefore she should be reassured.

Myerson SG et al., *Emergencies in Cardiology*, Second Edition, Oxford University Press, 2010, Chapter 5, Palpitation, Diagnosing palpitation.

4. C. Gadolinium enhancement on cardiac magnetic resonance imaging

Although gadolinium enhancement on CMR in hypertrophic cardiomyopathy has been shown to confer a worse prognosis, it is not a conventional risk factor under current guidelines to mandate implantation of an ICD for primary prophylaxis of sudden cardiac death.

Maron BJ et al., Task Force on Clinical Expert Consensus Documents. American College of Cardiology; Committee for Practice Guidelines. European Society of Cardiology, *Journal of the American College of Cardiology* 2003;42(9):1687–1713.

5. C. Implantable cardioverter defibrillator

This patient is at very high risk of sudden death due to a ventricular arrhythmia. Whilst myomectomy may impact on symptoms of angina or syncope, it does not reduce the risk of ventricular tachycardia. As such an implantable cardioverter defibrillator is the most appropriate option. If he refuses this device then regular amiodarone would be a potential alternative.

Ramrakha P, Hill J, *Oxford Handbook of Cardiology*, First Edition, Oxford University Press, 2006, Chapter 11, Invasive electrophysiology, Automatic implantable cardioverter defibrillators.

6. D. Lengthening PR interval

The increasing PR interval raises the possibility of extension of the infection into the myocardium. It may be suggestive of myocardial abscess formation. Other indications for surgery include septal perforation and valvular obstruction, and severe mitral or aortic regurgitation. Depending on the defect surgery may be targeted at removal/debridement of infected tissue or valve replacement.

Longmore M et al., *Oxford Handbook of Clinical Medicine*, Eighth Edition, Oxford University Press, 2010.

7. D. LDH

LDH is the last enzyme to rise after myocardial infarction, beginning its rise 2–5 days after MI and remaining elevated for around 10 days afterwards. GPBB becomes elevated 1–3 hours after myocardial infarction and is therefore the earliest biochemical marker of infarction. LDH is the last enzyme to rise after myocardial infarction, beginning its rise 2–5 days after MI and remaining elevated for around 10 days afterwards. CK is elevated 6 hours after infarction, but specific isoenzyme measurement is required to determine that the rise is due to cardiac muscle damage. Conventional practice in the UK is to measure 6 and 12-hour troponin levels to establish biochemical evidence of myocardial damage; this is because the assay is reliable and sensitive with respect to very low levels of cardiac muscle damage, and any rise can be seen by 12 hours after the onset of chest pain.

Ramrakha P, Hill J, *Oxford Handbook of Cardiology*, First Edition, Oxford University Press, 2006, Chapter 5, Coronary artery disease, STEM1: diagnosis.

8. E. Warfarin

Given moderate left atrial enlargement and a history of previous ischaemic heart disease, warfarinization is most appropriate for this patient to reduce her risk of embolic stroke. INR target should be 2–3. Other risk factors for embolic disease include left ventricular failure and a previous history of stroke or TIA. On CHADS VASC scoring she merits a score of 2, which helps to support the rationale for anti-coagulation in permanent AF.

Ramrakha P, Hill J, *Oxford Handbook of Cardiology*, First Edition, Oxford University Press, 2006, Chapter 10, Arrhythmias, Atrial fibrillation: management.

9. C. Left bundle branch block

Causes of reversed splitting of the second heart sound include left bundle branch block, aortic stenosis, and hypertrophic obstructive cardiomyopathy. Fixed splitting of the second heart sound where there is no variance with respiration occurs in the presence of an ASD or VSD.

Ramrakha P, Hill J, *Oxford Handbook of Cardiology*, First Edition, Oxford University Press, 2006, Chapter 10, Arrhythmias, Bundle branch block.

10. B. Amiodarone and magnesium

This patient has monomorphic ventricular tachycardia but with preserved blood pressure. As such, correction of electrolyte imbalance and attempted IV cardioversion is reasonable. The magnesium is less than 1.0, as such magnesium infusion is acceptable, as is IV amiodarone. Sotolol or procainamide are reasonable alternatives. Ambulatory ECG monitoring/referral to a cardiac electrophysiologist is advised to decide on long-term management.

Ramrakha P et al., *Oxford Handbook of Acute Medicine*, Third Edition, Oxford University Press, 2010.

11. B. Clopidogrel 300 mg

The ECG appearance is consistent with NSTEMI, and given his history of type 2 diabetes and smoking, he is at significant risk of a further event. As such they should be managed with both high-dose aspirin and 300 mg of clopidgrel. He should also be given fondaparinux (NICE CG94). Nitrates or diamorphine could be considered for patients with ongoing pain. Whilst NICE technology assessment of ticagrelor recommends its use for NSTEMIs, NICE guidance on coronary artery syndromes still recommends clopidogrel. No doubt this inconsistency will be corrected before too long.

Ramrakha P et al., *Oxford Handbook of Acute Medicine*, Third Edition, Oxford University Press, 2010.

12. C. Ramipril

Ramipril is an ACEI. This can cause problems with foetal and neonatal blood pressure control if used during pregnancy. It can also cause renal failure in the foetus and other abnormalities such as oligohydramnios. Methyldopa is often used in pregnancy to control blood pressure, as is Nifedipine. Hydralazine may be used IV to treat uncontrolled BP in an acute situation, as may Labetolol.

British National Formulary, 2 Cardiovascular system, https://www.evidence.nhs.uk/formulary/bnf/current/2-cardiovascular-system

13. B. Coxsackie virus

The symptoms here are consistent with myocarditis, of which Coxsackie virus is the commonest recognized viral cause. It also occurs in a number of inflammatory conditions such as sarcoidosis and SLE. Treatment is supportive, with standard medications for heart failure such as ACE inhibitors and diuretics. Patients are recommended to reduce their physical activity, sometimes for a number of months post diagnosis.

Torok E et al., *Oxford Handbook of Infectious Diseases and Microbiology*, Oxford University Press, 2009.

14. D. Imaging confirms pericardial calcification

Pericardial calcification on CXR or CT is characteristic of constrictive pericardial disease. Constrictive physiology is more strongly associated with a peak early velocity of expansion of greater than 8 cm s^{-1} and normal myocardial systolic contractility. Restrictive cardiomyopathy is more likely present if there is a pressure difference of greater than 6 mmHg between the left and right end diastolic pressures, and pulmonary artery pressures are greater than 50 mmHg.

Ramrakha P, Hill J, *Oxford Handbook of Cardiology*, First Edition, Oxford University Press, 2006, Chapter 9, Pericardial diseases.

15. C. *PRKAR1A* gene mutations

PRKAR1A mutations cause the Carney syndrome or complex. The myxomatous tumours that proliferate in Carney syndrome affect the heart, skin, breasts, pituitary, and testes among other tissues. Atrial myxomas are more likely to be bilateral and recur after surgery than in sporadic cases. Transmission is autosomal dominant and the condition tends to affect patients in their third decade of life. CK transporter mutations cause childhood intellectual impairment and myopathy. Incomplete penetrance and genetic anticipation are not features of the condition.

Ramrakha P, Hill J, *Oxford Handbook of Cardiology*, First Edition, Oxford University Press, 2006, Chapter 16, Eponymous syndromes.

16. A. Brugada syndrome

This ECG is classical of Brugada syndrome, as is the history with nocturnal attacks in a male and a positive family history. CPVT usually occurs on exercise and the ECG is generally normal; the QT interval is not prolonged, making any form of long QT syndrome much less likely, and right ventricular dysplasia can cause T wave abnormalities in V1 to V3, but does not cause right bundle branch block. AVSD can cause incomplete RBBB and left axis deviation, but does not explain the history.

Benito B et al., Brugada syndrome, *Progress in Cardiovascular Diseases* 2008;51(1):1–22.

17. C. Pre-excited atrial fibrillation

This rhythm shows a rapid tachycardia with prolonged QRS complexes, however careful inspection shows that the RR intervals are irregularly irregular, making this some form of atrial fibrillation. In a young woman, rate related aberration is less likely and furthermore, some of the broadest QRS complexes are associated with longer, rather than shorter, RR intervals. This ECG is therefore typical of pre-excited atrial fibrillation in someone with Wolff–Parkinson–White syndrome.

Ramrakha P, Hill J, *Oxford Handbook of Cardiology*, First Edition, Oxford University Press, 2006.

18. D. Eplerenone

Eplerenone is indicated post myocardial infarction in those with impaired systolic function and symptoms or signs of heart failure. Two weeks post MI is within the licensed indication period, and in the Ephesus study this medication was shown to have significant prognostic benefit. Digoxin has been shown to have only symptomatic benefit, not prognostic, and likewise there is no clear evidence for adding an ARB to a reasonable dose of an ACE inhibitor. Biventricular pacing does have prognostic benefit, but is only indicated once a patient has been established for a period on full appropriate medical therapy, which is not yet the case with this patient. Ivabradine has also recently been shown to have prognostic benefit in the SHIFT study, but does not yet have a licence for this indication and an entry criterion for the study was a heart rate over 70.

SHIFT study: Swedberg K, Komajda M, Böhm M, et al., SHIFT investigators, ivabradine and outcomes in chronic heart failure (SHIFT): a randomised placebo-controlled study, *Lancet* 2010;376(9744):875–885.

19. E. Left ventricular hypertrophy

The M mode line is taken across the left ventricle in the parasternal long axis view. There is marked symmetrical left ventricular thickening (diastolic thickness around 2 cm, septum and posterior walls are equally affected). In addition the left ventricular systolic function is very good. Hypertrophic cardiomyopathy typically preferentially affects the septum and amyloidosis, although it can cause hypertrophy, and is also associated with ventricular dilatation and poor LV function. Fabry's disease is rare, although it can cause ventricular wall thickening, and Kearns–Sayres syndrome (a mitochondrial myopathy) is very rare and not associated with LVH. This leaves LVH as the correct diagnosis.

Ramrakha P, Hill J, *Oxford Handbook of Cardiology*, First Edition, Oxford University Press, 2006.

20. B. Beta blocker and warfarin

The initial priorities in management of symptomatic, but haemodynamically stable atrial fibrillation are rate control, which is best done with a beta blocker and risk assessment for thrombo-embolic complications. Digoxin is commonly used, but rarely controls the heart rate, particularly on exercise, and should not be first line. This man's CHADS2 score is 3 (age, hypertension, and echo evidence of structural heart disease); he thus has an annual risk of thrombo-embolic complications of around 6%, so should be formally anticoagulated and not just given aspirin.

NICE, The management of atrial fibrillation—CG36. https://www.nice.org.uk/guidance/cg36.

21. D. Ivabradine

The principal goal in the symptomatic management of those with angina should be to get the heart rate under 60, or under 55 in those with severe angina. This is frequently not achieved with a beta blocker alone, even when the beta blocker is appropriately up-titrated, which is frequently not the case. An ACE inhibitor has prognostic advantage in those with vascular disease but no symptomatic benefit in this case and while both surgery and PCI are very effective symptomatic treatments, medical therapy should normally be optimized first before offering invasive treatment. Ivabradine can be added to a beta blocker and is effective both in controlling the heart rate and also in improving anginal symptoms.

BEAUTIFUL study: Fox K, Ford I, Steg PG et al., BEAUTIFUL investigators, ivabradine for patients with stable coronary artery disease and left-ventricular systolic dysfunction (BEAUTIFUL): a randomised, double-blind, placebo-controlled trial. *European Heart Journal* 2013 Aug;34(29):2263–2270. doi: 10.1093/eurheartj/eht101. Epub 2013 Mar 26.

22. D. Lisinopril

ACE inhibitors have been shown to have benefits in patients with vascular disease without LV dysfunction, in a number of studies (reviewed in the reference given here). In stable angina, as opposed to acute coronary syndromes, PCI has never been shown to be of any prognostic benefit. This has been shown repeatedly although the latest and best known trial is the COURAGE study.

Jolliffe JA et al., Exercise-based rehabilitation for coronary heart disease, *Cochrane Database of Systematic Reviews* 2000;(4):CD001800. Review UPDATE in: *Cochrane database of systematic reviews* 2001.

23. E. The tips of the valves are preferentially affected but the inflammatory process

Erythema marginatum is a major criterion in the diagnosis of rheumatic fever, not erythema nodosum. Globally the disease is still common, although it has become quite rare (although not unknown) in the West and is caused by a group A streptococcus. Typically it takes several years after the initial acute rheumatic fever before the carditis produces sufficient valvular disease for symptoms to occur.

Cilliers AM, Rheumatic fever and its management, *British Medical Journal* 2006;333:1153.

24. B. Coronary calcium score

This is a low-risk patient presenting with atypical cardiac pain and, based on the new NICE guidance for the investigation of chest pain, a coronary calcium score is the most appropriate investigation. Note that exercise testing is not recommended at all for the investigation of chest pain in the latest NICE guidance.

CG 95. Chest pain of recent onset. Assessment and diagnosis of recent onset chest pain or discomfort of suspected cardiac origin. https://www.nice.org.uk/guidance/cg95/chapter/Introduction.

25. A. Abundant neutrophils

Abundant lymphocytes and tissue monocytes are features of highly inflamed, unstable atherosclerotic plaques, as are the features B to B, but neutrophils are not generally seen.

Ross R, Atherosclerosis: an inflammatory disease, *New England Journal of Medicine* 1999;340:115–126.

26. C. Dihydopyridine calcium antagonist

Although the BP is not very high, the presence of evidence of end-organ damage in the form of LVH suggests that the most recently endorsed target of <140/90 mmHg is appropriate. The NICE publication on the management of hypertension in primary care recommends that after an ACE inhibitor/ARB and thiazide, the next step in management should be a dihydropyridine calcium antagonist. This is followed by an alpha blocker, and beta blockers are only recommended fourth line. Spironolactone in very useful in hypertension associated with Conn's syndrome, but the high/normal potassium makes this very unlikely.

NICE clinical guideline 127. http://www.nice.org.uk/nicemedia/live/13561/56008/56008.pdf.

27. E. Tachycardia

The commonest physical signs in patients with tamponade are firstly tachycardia and a raised JVP, later with Kussmaul's sign, hypotension, and finally signs of low cardiac output. Although mentioned in all the books, cardiac dullness beyond the apex beat is rarely detectable. One would not expect to hear a pericardial rub because fluid is separating the two layers of the pericardium and the steep y descent of the JVP (Friedrich's sign) is more typical of constrictive pericarditis.

Ramrakha P, Hill J, *Oxford Handbook of Cardiology*, Oxford University Press, 2006, Chapter 9, Pericardial diseases.

28. B. Cessation of alcohol

In contrast to other forms of cardiomyopathy, the prognosis can be massively improved by cessation of alcohol. Of course, other interventions such as beta blockade, ACE inhibition, and spironolactone may also impact on prognosis, but by far the biggest impact is gained by alcohol cessation. Symptoms may drastically improve or even resolve in some cases over a period of a few months.

Ramrakha P, Hill J, *Oxford Handbook of Cardiology*, First Edition, Oxford University Press, 2006, Chapter 8, Heart muscle diseases, Alcoholic cardiomyopathy.

29. D. Imaging confirms pericardial calcification

Pericardial calcification on CXR or CT is characteristic of constrictive pericardial disease. Constrictive physiology is more strongly associated with a peak early velocity of expansion of greater than 8 cm s^{-1} and normal myocardial systolic contractility. Restrictive cardiomyopathy is more likely present if there is a pressure difference of greater than 6 mmHg between the left and right end diastolic pressures and pulmonary artery pressures are greater than 50 mmHg.

Ramrakha P, Hill J, *Oxford Handbook of Cardiology*, First Edition, Oxford University Press, 2006, Chapter 9, Pericardial diseases.

30. B. Intracardiac shunting increases with age due to increasing left ventricular stiffness

Intracardiac shunting increases with age due to increasing left ventricular stiffness. This is an important clinical phenomenon since there is an associated increased risk of atrial arrhythmias and pulmonary hypertension. Closure is indicated in all symptomatic patients without specific age limits. Sinus venosus and partial atrio-ventricular septal defects require surgical closure. Endocarditis is rare and antibiotic prophylaxis is not indicated.

Ramrakha P, Hill J, *Oxford Handbook of Cardiology*, First Edition, Oxford University Press, 2006, Chapter 12, Congenital heart disease.

31. A. Amyloidosis

Whilst formerly secondary amyloidosis used to complicate chronic infections (e.g. chronic empyema or osteomyelitis), more commonly it now complicates chronic inflammatory disorders, include ankylosing spondylitis, chronic rheumatoid arthritis, and psoriatic arthropathy. Cardiac involvement may be suspected by echocardiography but a SAP scan will detect the extent of the disease. Libman–Sachs endocarditis is associated with systemic lupus erythematosus. Haemochromatosis may be associated with cardiac failure but renal involvement is not characteristic although any patient with severe right-sided heart failure may develop some proteinuria.

Ramrakha P, Hill J, *Oxford Handbook of Cardiology*, First Edition, Oxford University Press, 2006, Chapter 13, Multisystem disorders.

32. D. Bisoprolol

This patient has ischaemic heart disease, left atrial enlargement, and LV dysfunction. As such, bisoprolol is the most appropriate option. As well as giving rate control, it has been shown in heart failure to have a positive impact on heart failure, with outcome benefits seen in the CIBIS 2 study. Carvedilol has similar outcome data to bisoprolol in heart failure.

Roy D et al., Rhythm control versus rate control for atrial fibrillation and heart failure, *New England Journal of Medicine* 2008;358:2667–2677. http://www.nejm.org/doi/full/10.1056/NEJMoa0708789.

33. D. Ruptured chordae tendinae

A relatively rare complication of myocardial infarction is rupture of the chordae tendinae of the mitral valve, resulting in a pansystolic murmur. However, one needs to be aware of the condition as it causes sudden deterioration in a patient's condition. Partial or complete rupture occurs 2–5 days post infarct. It may result in cardiogenic shock and acute pulmonary oedema and emergency surgery is necessary. Cardiogenic shock characteristically presents with the acute infarct. The possibility of a further infarct should be considered but the presence of a new murmur points to the diagnosis. Pericarditis, or Dressler's syndrome, may occur in up to 20% of patients in the week following a myocardial infarct, but presents with pain.

Warrell DA et al., *Oxford Textbook of Medicine*, Fifth Edition, Oxford University Press, 2010, Section 16.6, Heart valve disease.

34. B. Myotonic dystrophy

Myotonic dystrophy is not associated with restrictive cardiomyopathy. The remaining conditions are associated with restrictive cardiomyopathy: scleroderma (non-infiltrative cardiomyopathy), sarcoidosis and amyloidosis (infiltrative), Fabry's (metabolic), and haemochromatosis (Fe storage disease).

Ramrakha P, Hill J, *Oxford Handbook of Cardiology*, First Edition, Oxford University Press, 2006, Chapter 8, Heart muscle diseases.

35. E. Persistent left ventricular dilation

Persistent left ventricular dilation is not itself an indication for revision surgery, as ventricular remodelling may occur over time or be due to alternative causes of cardiomyopathy. Correct indications for mitral valve revision surgery include persistent mitral regurgitation (Grade 2+), persistent LVOT obstruction, mitral stenosis (mean gradient >6 mmHg, MVA <1/5 cm²), and leaflet perforation.

Ramrakha P, Hill J, *Oxford Handbook of Cardiology*, First Edition, Oxford University Press, 2006, Chapter 1, Cardiac investigations.

36. D. Is more commonly associated with aortic regurgitation than mitral regurgitation

Aortic regurgitation is one of the most common cardiovascular complications of ankylosing spondylitis (1–10%) while mitral valve regurgitation is much rarer, despite occasional mitral valve thickening. Aortitis is also common, causing dilatation rather than constriction of the ascending aorta (C). Ankylosing spondylitis affects 1–2% of HLA B-27-positive individuals (A) and is three times more common in males (B). It is not frequently associated with early onset coronary disease, but has been reported to cause coronary artery aneurysms.

Ramrakha P, Hill J, *Oxford Handbook of Cardiology*, First Edition, Oxford University Press, 2006, Chapter 13, Multisystem disorders.

37. E. Not an indication for beta-blocker therapy

Brugada syndrome, an important cause of sudden cardiac death in young patients, is not an indication for beta-blocker therapy. The only proven treatment for Brugada syndrome is AICD implantation, although some evidence suggests quinidine may have some beneficial effects. Beta-blockers and amiodarone are associated with a high mortality in Brugada syndrome. Brugada syndrome inheritance is autosomal dominant. It is caused by *SCN5A* mutations. *KCNJ2* mutations cause K+ channelopathy Andersen Tawil Syndromes. Classical ECG changes include RBBB and ST elevations in V1-3. Procainamide and amjaline are used to diagnostically provoke, not treat, Brugada syndrome.

Brugada P, Brugada J, Right bundle branch block, persistent ST segment elevation and sudden cardiac death: a distinct clinical and electrocardiographic syndrome. A multicenter report, *Journal of the American College of Cardiology* 1992;20(6):1391–1396.

38. B. Spontaneous arterial rupture

Eighty percent of patients suffer a major arterial complication by the age of 40 years. Most deaths are caused by arterial rupture. Intestinal ruptures are common but usually less fatal. Uncontrolled bleeding from trauma has been reported but is not a major cause of death. Mitral valve prolapse and regurgitation is common but secondary cardiac failure is uncommon. Tissue healing is generally impaired but immunosuppression and infection are not characteristic features of the condition.

Germain DP, Clinical and genetic features of vascular Ehlers–Danlos syndrome, *Annals of Vascular Surgery* 2002;16:391–397.

39. B. Calcific degeneration of a bicuspid valve

Calcific degeneration of a bicuspid valve. Congenital bicuspid valve disease has a distinct epidemiology to acquired tricuspid disease, with an earlier onset of more severe disease more likely to lead to valve replacement and aortopathy. Furthermore, it is important to be aware of this pattern because bicuspid valves may have implications for family screening. Bicuspid valve disease represents ~50% of disease; tricuspid valve disease ~30–40%; and unicuspid disease ~10%. Rheumatic disease represents less than 20% of aortic valve disease in the UK. Metabolic derangements (hypercalcaemia, etc.) can cause aortic stenosis but are rare as an overall cause.

Camm AJ et al., *The ESC Textbook of Cardiovascular Medicine*, Second Edition, Oxford University Press, 2010, Chapter 21, Valvular heart disease.

40. E. Right ventricular outflow tract

The ECG has a left bundle branch block pattern, indicating that it arises from the right heart so only answer D or E are viable. The heart's electrical axis refers to the general direction of the depolarization wavefront in the frontal plane. With a healthy conducting system the cardiac axis is related to where the major muscle bulk of the heart lies. Normally, this is the left ventricle with some contribution from the right ventricle. Values of −30° to +90° are considered to be normal. If the left ventricle increases its activity or bulk then there is said to be 'left axis deviation' as the axis swings round to the left beyond −30°; alternatively in conditions where the right ventricle is strained or hypertrophied then the axis swings round beyond +90° and 'right axis deviation' is said to exist. Disorders of the conduction system of the heart (in this case ventricular tachycardia) can disturb the electrical axis without necessarily reflecting changes in muscle bulk. Here the axis is positive in the inferior leads, indicating superior to inferior travel of depolarization. The only remaining anatomical choices are right ventricular outflow tract (superior location) and right ventricular apex (inferior location), hence overall the origin is most likely to be from the right ventricular outflow tract.

Segal OR et al., A novel algorithm for determining endocardial VT exit site from 12-lead surface ECG characteristics in human, infarct-related ventricular tachycardia, *Journal of Cardiovascular Electrophysiology* 2007;18:161–168. http://onlinelibrary.wiley.com/doi/10.1111/j.1540-8167.2007.00721.x/full.

41. A. Bisoprolol

The management of HCM includes negative inotropes such as beta-blockers and verapamil. In the case of heart failure symptoms, beta-blockers are the initial drug of choice. ACE inhibitors may actually worsen symptoms when there is significant outflow tract obstruction. Myomectomy is reserved for patients who fail medical therapy. Amiodaraone may be used to control arrhythmias, although if there is documented VT, patients progress to an implantable cardioverter defibrillator. Positive inotropes such as digoxin are generally avoided, as they can exacerbate heart failure symptoms in the majority of patients with preserved LV function.

2014 ESC Guidelines on diagnosis and management of hypertrophic cardiomyopathy. *European Heart Journal* 2014; 35: 2733–2779.

42. A. Atrial flutter with 2:1 atrioventricular block

Adenosine will temporarily block conduction in the atrio-ventricular node. In the context of atrial flutter this will aid diagnosis by revealing atrial flutter waves but is unlikely to terminate the arrhythmia. Atrioventricular nodal re-entry tachycardia is a re-entry circuit within the AV node which is terminated by adenosine. Orthodromic atrioventricular re-entry tachycardia is not wholly confined to the AV node but can be terminated by adenosine in the same way. Catecholamine-sensitive ventricular tachycardia occurs in young people with structurally normal hearts. They are prone to exercise-induced ventricular tachycardia which is responsive to adenosine. Sinus node re-entry tachycardia may be sensitive to adenosine termination.

Garratt CJ et al., Adenosine and cardiac arrhythmias, *British Medical Journal* 1992;305(6844):3–4.

43. B. Sinus venosus defects may occur near the orifice of the inferior vena cava

Sinus venosus type defects can occur near the inferior or superior vena cava. They are often associated with anomalous venous drainage from the right lung. Fixed splitting occurs with an atrial septal defect. Secundum defects are true communications between the left and right atria, with flow between chambers. A patent foramen ovale is a normal variant with only a virtual space between atria. Primum defects are more common in Down's syndrome. The ECG shows right bundle branch block with left axis deviation in primum type defects.

Warnes CA et al., ACC/AHA 2008 guidelines for the management of adults with congenital heart disease: a report of the American College of Cardiology/American Heart Association Task Force on Practice Guidelines.

44. C. Patients with infective endocarditis complicated by locally uncontrolled infection, e.g. abscess formation

Patients with infective endocarditis complicated by locally uncontrolled infection, e.g. abscess formation: Level of evidence: I B. Coronary disease per se does not influence the level of recommendation for an operation, although it will increase the risk of surgery. Patients with infective endocarditis and no heart failure symptoms: Level of evidence IIa B. Patients with vegetations >10 mm and signs of heart failure: Level of evidence: I C. atients with very large vegetations (in excess of 15 mm): Evidence class IIb level C.

ESC guidelines on Infective Endocarditis, https://www.escardio. org/Guidelines-&-Education/Clinical-Practice-Guidelines/ Infective-Endocarditis-Guidelines-on-Prevention-Diagnosis-and-Treatment-of.

45. C. Arrhythmogenic right ventricular cardiomyopathy

The epsilon wave is a major criterion in the diagnosis of arrhythmogenic right ventricular cardiomyopathy, a rare inherited cardiomyopathy that is characterized by cardiac fibrofatty infiltration and arrhythmias. The epsilon wave is a terminal notching of the QRS complex in the right praecordial leads, seen in approximately 30% of patients. Other ECG findings may include T-wave inversion, right bundle branch block, and prolongation of the right praecordial QRS complex, and late potentials may be recorded on signal averaged ECG. Frequent ventricular ectopics and non-sustained VT may be captured on a Holter monitor.

Basso C et al., Arrhythmogenic right ventricular cardiomyopathy, *Lancet* 2009;373(9671):1289–1300.

46. D. Long QT syndrome type 1

The diagnosis is long QT syndrome type 1. LQT1 accounts for roughly 50% of cases of LQTS and occurs due to mutations in the KCNQ1 gene. In LQT1, exercise, particularly swimming, is a classic trigger for development of arrhythmias. In LQT2 syndrome, adrenergic stress or loud noise may trigger arrhythmia. Brugada syndrome is an inherited arrhythmia syndrome due to mutations in *SCN5A*, most commonly found in Southeast Asian males.

Schwartz PJ et al., Genotype–phenotype correlation in the long-QT syndrome: gene-specific triggers for life-threatening arrhythmias, *Circulation* 2001;103;89–95.

47. E. The most common organism in fungal endocarditis is Candida species

Candida is the most common cause of fungal infective endocarditis. Other common fungal causes include histoplasmosis and aspergillosis. A is incorrect—fungal infective endocarditis is more common in patients with prosthetic valves or a history of injecting drug use. D is incorrect—mortality rates from fungal infective endocarditis are usually greater than 50%. B is incorrect—fungal infective endocarditis is commonly associated with bulky vegetations. C is incorrect—negative serology and cultures are often negative in fungal infective endocarditis.

Ramrakha P, Hill J, *Oxford Handbook of Cardiology*, First Edition, Oxford University Press, 2006, Chapter 4, Infective endocarditis.

48. A. Acute mitral valve rupture

This patient has suffered an inferior myocardial infarction and the symptoms are most consistent with acute mitral valve rupture. Complete valvular rupture causes torrential MR and is invariably fatal. In inferior MI valvular rupture is usually due to posteromedial papillary muscle rupture. The diagnosis is confirmed by echocardiography. Where blood pressure allows, treatment with vasodilators is the initial therapy of choice, with early surgical review to determine the possibility of surgical intervention.

Ramrakha P et al., *Oxford Handbook of Acute Medicine*, Third Edition, Oxford University Press, 2010.

49. C. Dressler's syndrome

Dressler's syndrome is an autoimmune pericarditis following a myocardial infarct. A similar clinical picture may complicate cardiac surgery and is termed post-cardiomyotomy syndrome. Clinical features include a low-grade fever and a pericardial friction rub. It is usually self-limiting but may respond to NSAIDs or (if needed) steroids.

Longmore M et al., *Oxford Handbook of Clinical Medicine*, Eighth Edition, Oxford University Press, 2010, Chapter 3, Cardiovascular medicine, Complications of MI.

50. C. Myotonic dystrophy with second degree heart block

Conduction problems are common following myocardial infarction, particularly when involving the right coronary artery as it supplies the cardiac nodal and conduction tissue. Many arrhythmias are therefore transitory, and will resolve in the days following an infarct. If a patient is haemodynamically compromised, consideration should be paid to temporary cardiac pacing. Permanent pacing is therefore not a class I indication immediately following a myocardial infarction, but may become so depending on the recovery of the conducting system.

Vardas PE et al., Guidelines for cardiac pacing and cardiac resynchronisation therapy. The task force for cardiac pacing and cardiac resynchronisation therapy of the European Society of Cardiology. Developed in collaboration with the European Heart Rhythm.

51. D. Percutaneous drainage of the pericardial effusion

Radiation pericarditis may occur during or immediately following treatment, but it is more usually delayed for more than 12 months. Pericardial fibrosis is a common cause of effusions and often requires drainage in approximately 50% of patients with pericardial effusions. Radiation pericarditis is dependent on radiation field, dose, duration, malignancy type (breast and lymphoma), and patient age. Lung and coronary artery radation damage are rare and pulmonary emboli are unlikely after 18 months.

Ramrakha P, Hill J, *Oxford Handbook of Cardiology*, First Edition, Oxford University Press, 2006, Chapter 3, Cardiovascular medicine, Pericardial diseases.

52. E. Transthoracic echocardiogram

This ECG is classical for the apical form of hypertrophic cardiomyopathy. A transthoracic echocardiogram will confirm the diagnosis in the majority of cases and is quick, cheap, and non-invasive. A coronary angiogram may need to be performed at some stage but should not be the initial investigation, particularly after a two-day history of chest pain. In cases where transthoracic echocardiography fails to make the diagnosis, a CMR is often useful. Cardiac troponin levels can be measured to help exclude a coronary event, but will not confirm the diagnosis. There is no indication to perform a thoracic CT scan given the clinical scenario at present.

Yamaguchi H et al., Hypertrophic nonobstructive cardiomyopathy with giant negative T waves (apical hypertrophy): ventriculographic and echocardiographic features in 30 patients, *American Journal of Cardiology* 1979;44(3):401–412.

53. B. Splenomegaly

Whilst the most common cause of hypertension is idiopathic, it is important to consider other causes, such as renal artery stenosis (small kidney), phaeochromocytoma (adrenal mass), and adult polycystic kidney disease. Aortic calcification is likely to relate to atherosclerosis, a risk factor for which is hypertension. Splenomegaly is seen in portal hypertension as opposed to systemic.

Dahnert W, *Radiology Review Manual*, Fifth Edition, Lippincott Williams & Wilkins, 2003, Urogenital disorders, p. 869.

54. B. Clarithromycin

The ECG shows prolongation of the QT interval. Patients with undiagnosed long QT syndrome are at risk of developing torsade de pointes with drugs including macrolide antibiotics such as clarithromycin.

Drugs to be avoided in patients with long QT syndrome: Focus on the anaesthesiological management, *World Journal of Cardiology* 2013 Apr 26;5(4):87–93.

55. C. Add warfarin

This man may be breathless for a number of reasons which should be investigated accordingly. However, he has atrial fibrillation with hypertension, age >75 and has had a previous TIA. His CHADS 2 score is 4. He is on no thromboprophylactic medication and it is therefore a priority to discuss formal anticoagulation with the patient, and ideally commence warfarin.

European Heart Rhythm Association et al., Guidelines for the management of atrial fibrillation: the Task Force for the Management of Atrial Fibrillation of the European Society of Cardiology (ESC).

56. A. Carotid sinus massage

It is entirely reasonable in the presence of preserved blood pressure to try vagal manoeuvres first, before progressing to drug therapy. If drug therapy is required, however, a range of calcium antagonists is a reasonable option. Swallowing crushed ice, or carotid sinus massage, are both potential vagal stimulation techniques. If the patient's blood pressure was significantly compromised, then electrical cardioversion would be the intervention of choice. Recurrent tachycardias may be managed with ablation therapy. He should of course be told not to abuse cocaine again.

Katritsis M, Camm J, Contemporary reviews in cardiovascular medicine: atrioventricular nodal reentrant tachycardia, *Circulation* 2010;122:831–840. http://circ.ahajournals.org/cgi/content/extract/122/8/831.

57. A. Pulmonary stenosis

All the abnormalities except pulmonary stenosis cause a reversed split of the second heart sound. Pulmonary stenosis results in a widely split second heart sound.

Kalra PA, *Essential Revision Notes for MRCP*, Third Edition, PasTest, 2009, Chapter 1, Cardiology, Heart sounds, p. 5.

58. E. It should be administered at high doses for at least one month before slow tapering

If indicated, steroid therapy should be administered at high doses with slow tapering to minimize the risk of disease recurrence. The COlchicine in addition to conventional therapy for acute PEricarditis (COPE) trial found that early administration of steroids for acute pericarditis was associated with an increased incidence of relapse after steroid weaning. Indeed, steroid use was an independent predictor of relapse (odds ratio 4:3). Steroids administered concurrently with colchicine is also a risk factor for disease recurrence. It is therefore recommended that steroids be used in patients unresponsive to NSAIDs or colchicine. Intrapericardial steroid therapy is more invasive but not associated with the risk of recurrence found with oral steroid therapy.

Imazio M et al., Colchicine in addition to conventional therapy for acute pericarditis: results of the COlchicine for acute PEricarditis (COPE) trial, *Circulation* 2005;112(13):2012–2016.

59. B. Type 2 MI

The question clearly describes a woman who is septic secondary to pneumonia. Her condition is complicated by atrial fibrillation with fast ventricular response (160 bpm). At such fast rates it is not uncommon for resting ECGs to reveal marked ischaemia, particularly in elderly patients. The blood tests that have been performed have revealed a grossly elevated troponin, and in association with an ischaemic ECG this raises the possibility of a myocardial infarct. The crux of the question here is whether or not the infarct is secondary to a type 1 MI (ischaemia due to a primary coronary event, such as plaque erosion and/or rupture, fissuring, or dissection) or a type 2 MI (as a consequence of impaired myocardial blood supply, due in this case to the tachyarrhythmia and hypotension). The latter option is the most likely in this patient. Importantly aggressive anticoagulation is not indicated in this setting. The other classes of MI are as follows: type 3—sudden unexpected cardiac death, including cardiac arrest, often with symptoms suggesting ischaemia with new ST-segment elevation; new left bundle branch block; or pathologic or angiographic evidence of fresh coronary thrombus— in the absence of reliable biomarker findings; type 4a—MI associated with PCI; type 4b—MI associated with documented in-stent thrombosis; type 5 MI—associated with CABG surgery.

Thygesen K et al., Universal definition of myocardial infarction, *Circulation* 2007;116:2634–2653.

60. C. No change in blood pressure during exercise tolerance testing

Hypertrophic cardiomyopathy risk stratification is a clinically important and well established basis for ICD implantation. The major risk factors documented in the current ACC/AHA/HRS guidance for device-based therapy are: prior cardiac arrest, spontaneous sustained or non-sustained VT, family history of sudden cardiac death, syncope, LV wall thickness >30 mm, and abnormal blood pressure response to exercise.

Priori SG et al., Task force on sudden cardiac death of the European Society of Cardiology, *European Heart Journal* 2001;22:1374.

61. A. They are contraindicated in constrictive pericarditis

Glyceryl trinitrate sublingual sprays are used to relieve the chest pain in anterior myocardial infarction but nitrates aggravate the symptoms of HOCM by reducing the left ventricular volume. Having glaucoma is not a contraindication to receiving nitrates. Nitrates do not reduce the production of nitric oxide. Glyceryl trinitrate sublingual sprays are used to relieve the chest pain in anterior myocardial infarction but nitrates aggravate the symptoms of HOCM by reducing the left ventricular volume. A reduction in diastolic filling by nitrates causes a further reduction in cardiac output in patients with constrictive pericarditis.

Longmore M et al., *Oxford Handbook of Clinical Medicine*, Eighth Edition, Oxford University Press, 2010, Chapter 3, Cardiovascular medicine, Pericardial diseases.

62. B. Beta myosin heavy chain

Sarcomeric HCM is the commonest subtype of hypertophic cardiomyopathy, involving mutations in genes that encode proteins in the basic contractile unit of cardiac muscle: the sarcomere. More than a dozen different genes have been identified as potentially causative, with hundreds of different mutations. Of these, mutations in beta myosin heavy chain are the commonest.

Alcalai R et al., Genetic basis of hypertrophic cardiomyopathy: from bench to the clinics, *Journal of Cardiovascular Electrophysiology* 2008;19(1):104–110.

63. E. Ventricular septal defect

Ventricular septal defect is the commonest congenital heart condition and, particularly when small and thus haemodynamically insignificant, tends to cause a very loud, harsh systolic murmur, sometimes associated with a thrill (Maladie de Roger). The patient is well and not cyanosed, thus Fallot's is most unlikely as this is a cyanotic condition, although a loud systolic murmur may be present due to pulmonary infundibular stenosis. ASD can cause a systolic flow murmur, but this is rarely loud. Pulmonary atresia would need to be associated with a shunt to allow blood to get into the pulmonary circulation; thus, it is unlikely the patient would be entirely well and congenital aortic stenosis is much less common than VSD.

Penny DJ, Vick GW 3rd, Ventricular septal defect, *Lancet* 2011;377(9771):1103–1112.

64. C. Intravenous nitrates

This is a patient with acute heart failure and the hypertension shows that the afterload must be inappropriately high; thus the most effective treatment to improve cardiac output and reduce left ventricular filling pressures will be to reduce the afterload. This is best achieved with intravenous nitrates, although ACE inhibition would also be a reasonable option. Beta-blockade would not be first-line therapy in a patient with acute heart failure, and inotropes or balloon pumping are not indicated as the patient is hypertensive. Diuretics are not the best treatment, because the patient is in acute heart failure, thus is not likely to be salt and water overloaded from a whole-body point of view, but has fluid in the wrong place (in the form of pulmonary oedema) due to very high filling pressures due to inappropriately high afterload.

Cleland JGF et al., Acute heart failure: focusing on acute cardiogenic pulmonary oedema, *Clinical Medicine* 2010;10(1):59–64.

65. E. Primary pulmonary hypertension

Angina is very unlikely in a young woman of this age with no substantial risk factors. Much chest pain in this group would be benign, but this does not explain the collapses and abnormal ECG. Although the ECG could be superficially mistaken for right bundle branch block, in fact the QRS complexes are not wide enough for this and what is actually demonstrated is right ventricular hypertrophy, with a dominant R wave in V1, right axis deviation, and a narrow QRS complex (<0.12 s). Often there is also a deep S wave in V6, although not in this particular case. This is entirely consistent with pulmonary hypertension, and the history is also typical of primary pulmonary hypertension. The ECG is not consistent with either Brugada or long QT syndrome, which could cause collapses in a young woman (though Brugada syndrome is commoner in men), although neither of these is associated with chest pain or breathlessness. If pulmonary hypertension is confirmed, secondary causes should also be checked, such as HIV infection, connective tissue disease, or some drugs, such as anorexigens.

Archer SL, Michelakis ED, An evidence-based approach to the management of pulmonary arterial hypertension, *Current Opinion in Cardiology* 2006;21(4):385–392.

66. C. Fallot's tetralogy

The child clearly has some form of congenital heart disease and since he is cyanosed, this rules out congenitally corrected transposition and hypoplastic left heart, as neither of these cause cyanotic heart disease. ASD and VSD with Eisenmenger's are both possibilities, but shunt reversal at this early age would be most unlikely. Fallot's tetralogy is the commonest form of cyanotic congenital heart disease and the presence of the scar is consistent with the formation of a Blalock–Taussig shunt. This indicates that the condition must have given rise to severe obstruction of the outflow of the pulmonary side of the heart, necessitating the formation of a shunt, and again is consistent with the diagnosis of Fallot's.

Bhimji S, *Tetralogy of Fallot*, emedicine.medscape.com. http://emedicine.medscape.com/article/760387-overview.

67. C. Atrial septal defect (ASD)

Atrial septal defect (ASD) causes wide splitting of the second heart sound. This is due to increased flow through the pulmonary artery causing delayed pulmonary component of the second heart sound. Late A2 occurs in patients with left bundle branch block, aortic stenosis, and patent ductus arteriosus leading to paradoxical splitting of the second heart sound. Pulmonary embolism might be associated with loud P2 as a result of secondary pulmonary hypertension.

http://emedicine.medscape.com/article/162914-overview.

68. A. Diclofenac

The symptoms and ECG appearance are consistent with an underlying diagnosis of pericarditis. As such non-steroidal anti-inflammatories are appropriate with respect to pain relief. There is no indication for thrombolysis or angioplasty. The raised troponin potentially indicates an element of myocarditis. Uncomplicated cases do not require hospital admission. However, in view of the raised troponin, he should probably be advised not to undertake strenuous exercise. A pericardial rub is not invariably found, and ECG may be normal in 10%.

Myerson SG et al., *Emergencies in Cardiology*, Second Edition, Oxford University Press, 2010, Chapter 12, Pericardial disease, Pericarditis.

69. E. Refer for cardiac resynchronization therapy

This patient has NYHA class IV heart failure, and is on maximal therapy with an ACE inhibitor, spironolactone, and a selective beta-blocker. Given his blood pressure is only a little above 100 systolic, there is no room to further increase his oral medication. This leaves cardiac resynchronization therapy as the most appropriate option. This is effectively permanent dual chamber pacing, and is recommended by NICE guidelines for patients like this who have continued severe symptoms despite maximal tolerated medical therapy.

NICE guidelines: Cardiac resynchronisation therapy for the treatment of heart failure. http://www.nice.org.uk/TA120.

70. A. Add bisoprolol 2.5 mg

It is most appropriate in this case to add a beta-blocker licensed for the treatment of heart failure, the most appropriate choices being carvedilol or bisoprolol. Both are started at low dose and titrated to maximal tolerated dose. Spironolactone may also be added, but it is usually commenced at low dose, not 100 mg. Angiotensin receptor blockers may be added on top of ACE inhibitors but are usually reserved for patients who fail to respond to beta-blockade, and require careful monitoring of potassium.

Diagnosis and management of adults with chronic heart failure: summary of updated NICE guidance, *British Medical Journal* 2010;341:c4130. http://www.bmj.com/content/341/bmj.c4130.short?rss=1&cited-by=yes&legid=bmj;341/aug25_2/c4130.

71. A. Simple analgesia

It is obvious from the history that this man has suffered a significant chest injury, probably as a result of the seat belt/steering wheel impacting on his chest. Whilst the T-wave inversion and raised troponin may be consistent with ischaemia, given the proximity to his chest injury, the most likely cause is cardiac contusion. As such the most appropriate treatment is simple analgesia.

Kaye P, O'Sullivan I, Review: Myocardial contusion: emergency investigation and diagnosis, *Emergency Medicine Journal* 2002;19:8–10. http://emj.bmj.com/content/19/1/8.abstract.

72. A. Aortic valve replacement

The patient has severe symptomatic aortic stenosis. As such the optimal management is valve replacement, which has an operative mortality of approximately 1%.

Ramrakha P, Hill J, *Oxford Handbook of Cardiology*, First Edition, Oxford University Press, 2006, Chapter 3, Valvular heart disease, Aortic stenosis.

73. E. Surgical myomectomy

This patient has hypertrophic cardiomyopathy with obstruction and has marked symptoms due to left ventricular outflow tract obstruction. It is likely that his symptoms would be improved by myomectomy. Alcohol septal ablation may be considered an alternative to myomectomy. This does not however reduce the risk of rhythm disturbance and sudden cardiac death due to VT/VF. Risk of rhythm disturbance appears to be increased in patients with a septal thickness of >30 mmHg and these patients should be considered for implantable cardioverter defibrillator. This should be considered after surgical myomectomy because of the risk of peri-operative lead displacement or before alcohol septal ablation because of the risks of heart block and ventricular arrhythmias.

Mahboob A et al., Hypertrophic obstructive cardiomyopathy-alcohol septal ablation vs. myectomy: a meta-analysis, *European Heart Journal* 2009.

74. E. Tissue Doppler abnormalities on echocardiography

Tissue Doppler echocardiography is a contemporary echocardiographic tool that allows the measurement of intrinsic myocardial velocities. In restrictive cardiomyopathy, there is a reduction in left ventricular relaxation as a result of primary myocardial disease with a resultant decrease in tissue velocity. In contrast, in constrictive pericarditis, there is no significant myocardial dysfunction and tissue velocity is not decreased. Whilst calcification on a chest X-ray is more suggestive of constrictive cardiomyopathy, the diagnostic yield is low. Although equalization of diastolic pressure on catheterization is more common in constrictive cardiomyopathy, it does not exclude a restrictive process. Low voltages on ECG are relatively typical for both constrictive and restrictive cardiomyopathy. Kussmaul's sign may be positive in either condition, more commonly in constrictive pericarditis. It is not a reliable enough sign to accurately differentiate between the two.

ESC guidelines on Pericardial Diseases, https://www.escardio.org/Guidelines-&-Education/Clinical-Practice-Guidelines/Pericardial-Diseases-Guidelines-on-the-Diagnosis-and-Management-of.

75. B. Haemochromatosis

A number of clues in this case scenario include clinical signs of heart failure, hepatomegaly, small testes, and arthritis. The unifying cause of this is haemochromatosis which may cause a cardiomyopathy and hypogonadism as well as pseudo-gout due to pyrophosphate crystals. It should be noted that NSAIDs may precipitate heart failure as a result of salt and water retention in patients with heart disease who were previously stable.

Warrell DA et al., *Oxford Textbook of Medicine*, Fifth Edition, Oxford University Press, 2010, Section 12.7.1, Hereditary haemochromatosis.

76. D. Tricuspid regurgitation

All the above cardiac lesions are associated with systolic murmurs. A systolic murmur heard maximally at the lower left sternal edge raises the possibility of tricuspid regurgitation (TR). This valvular lesion is associated with giant 'v' waves seen in the jugular venous pressure waveform. These are essentially formed by merging of both 'a' and 'v' waves to form a large waveform. 'A' waves represent atrial systole and 'v' waves represent passive venous return to the right atrium with a closed tricuspid valve. In the presence of TR, blood leaks back from the right ventricle to the right atrium during ventricular systole. This increases both volume and hence pressure in the right atrium, producing a large waveform. The question describes the patient being an intravenous drug user and this should alert you to the possibility of infective endocarditis, which in such patients frequently affects the tricuspid valve.

http://www.blaufuss.org/.

77. A. Duchenne muscular dystrophy

Duchenne muscular dystrophy has the highest prevalence of dilated cardiomyopathy among these conditions. Most males with Duchenne muscular dystrophy, caused by severe dysfunction or absence of dystrophin, die before their third decade. As treatments for respiratory failure have improved (e.g. antibiotics and mechanical ventilation), many males with Duchenne muscular dystrophy are surviving respiratory failure to die from cardiac failure. Myotonic dystrophy typically causes heart block due to fibrofatty infiltration in the atrioventricular groove. Dilated cardiomyopathy is uncommon in myotonic dystrophy. Inclusion body myositis, myasthenia gravis, and limb girdle muscular dystrophy are not commonly associated with dilated cardiomyopathy. Duchenne muscular dystrophy is the commonest inherited myopathy affecting about 1:3500 live births. Candidates should be expected to know that respiratory failure and cardiac failure are important contributors to mortality in this condition.

Finsterer J, Stöllberger C, Cardiac involvement in primary myopathies, *Cardiology* 2000;94:1–11.

78. B. Viral myocarditis

The symptoms, signs, and troponin here are consistent with viral myocarditis, most likely to be related to Coxsackie B infection. Most cases of viral myocarditis are self-limiting, but the patient should be warned to reduce his training for a few days until he is completely recovered. ECHO cardiogram may show diffuse LV dysfunction. Other causes of viral myocarditis include CMV, dengue, hepatitis, EBV, varicella, and influenza.

Ramrakha P, Hill J, *Oxford Handbook of Cardiology*, First Edition, Oxford University Press, 2006, Chapter 8, Heart muscle diseases, Viral myocarditis.

79. D. Referral for consideration of colonoscopy

Streptococcus bovis bacteraemia or endocarditis has a strong association with underlying gastrointestinal malignancy, most commonly colonic. Culture of this organism should trigger clinicians to undertake endoscopic evaluation of the gastrointestinal tract. A TTE would be of use to assess valvular function in this patient but can be done at a later date.

Clincal review of infective endocarditis (diagnosis and management), *British Medical Journal* 2006;333. http://www.bmj.com/content/333/7563/334.

80. C. Adenosine

This patient has SVT and is symptomatic, but has no signs of instability. The ALS guidelines suggest that vagal manoeuvres should be attempted, and if this is not successful then adenosine should be given. Initially this is a 6 mg bolus, but a subsequent 12 mg bolus can be given if needed. The other medications listed are used for arrhythmias or cardiac arrests (adrenaline) but would not be the best choice here. Please refer to the ALS guidelines in the link provided for further information.

ALS Guidelines: Adult tachycardia algorithm. http://www.resus.org.uk/pages/glalgos.htm.

81. D. Adenosine

Adenosine is effective in cardioverting SVT, and has the advantage that it does not undergo significant transfer across the placenta. As such it is the most appropriate option here. Given this woman's advanced state of pregnancy, even a short anaesthetic for electrical cardioversion should be avoided if possible. Verapamil or short-acting beta-blocker would be second and third choices after adenosine in this patient.

Ramrakha P, Hill J, *Oxford Handbook of Cardiology*, First Edition, Oxford University Press, 2006, Chapter 15, Heart disease in pregnancy, Arrhythmias in pregnancy.

82. A. Atrial septal defect

Atrial septal defect leads to a fixed splitting of the second heart sound. Widely split second heart sound is a result of right bundle branch block, mitral regurgitation, deep inspiration, and pulmonary stenosis. Causes of a reversed splitting of the second heart sound include PDA, left bundle branch block, aortic stenosis, and right ventricular pacing. Causes of a single second heart sound include ventricular septal defect, pulmonary atresia, hypertension, Eisenmenger syndrome, and Tetralogy of Fallot.

Kalra PA, *Essential Revision Notes for MRCP*, Third Edition, PasTest, 2009, Chapter 1, Cardiology, Heart sounds, p. 5.

83. C. Aortic regurgitation

The history of previous dislocations raises the possibility of a connective tissue disorder such as Marfan's. Marfan's is associated with increased risk of acute aortic regurgitation, as the presentation with acute heart failure and a diastolic murmur suggests. Other causes include ascending aortic dissection and endocarditis. Definitive management is surgery, and the state of cardiac function at presentation is closely correlated with eventual outcome. Prior to surgery any pain should be managed with opiates, and fluid offloaded with furosemide if BP allows.

Keane MG, Pyeritz RE, Aortic diseases: medical management of Marfan syndrome, *Circulation* 2008;117:2802–2813.

84. A. *C. psittaci*

The most likely cause here of culture-negative endocarditis is *C. psittaci* caught from one of his birds, also the likely cause of his left lower lobe pneumonia. Whilst *S. viridans* is a common cause of initially 'culture-negative' endocarditis, we are not given any pointers in the history towards dental work or other foci of infection. Hence in the presence of bird keeping, it seems *C. psittaci* is more likely. Other causes of culture-negative endocarditis include *Brucella, Neisseria, Legionella, Mycobacteria*, the HACEK group of organisms, *rickettsiae*, and fungi.

Ramrakha P et al., *Oxford Handbook of Acute Medicine*, Third Edition, Oxford University Press, 2010, Q85 Answer.

85. E. IV diltiazem

This is a gentleman with a regular SVT at 150 bpm which should raise the possibility of atrial flutter with 2:1 block. Initial examination does not describe any 'red flag' symptoms (see link); therefore immediate DC cardioversion is not indicated. Initial attempts to slow/terminate the arrhythmia with vagal manoeuvres are unsuccessful. Carotid sinus massage should be used with caution in patients with previous stroke disease due to the risk of causing further emboli; if there are audible carotid bruits it is not advised. Resuscitation guidelines suggest the use of adenosine in such a patient. This short-lived naturally occurring purine nucleoside has an extremely short half life (<5 seconds) and temporarily blocks the AV node's conduction.

This can terminate re-entrant tachycardias or temporarily reveal atrial flutter waves whilst conduction is blocked. Adenosine is contraindicated in asthma as it can cause bronchospasm. Its use is also contraindicated in patients taking dipyridamole, as this drug can prolong the duration of AV blockade. Beta-blockers such as metoprolol would not be appropriate in this patient either, due to the risk of precipitating bronchospasm given his pre-existing asthma. Rate limitation with the calcium channel blocker is the most appropriate intervention from those listed above.

Adult Tachycardia Algorithm. Resus Council. https://www.resus.org.uk

86. D. Infective endocarditis

Main-line drug abusers are at risk of infective endocarditis, affecting the tricuspid valve. Besides the symptoms of infection, notably fever, anorexia, weight loss, rigors, and night sweats, patients experience the effects of infective emboli as well as manifestations of immune complex disease (i.e. microscopic haematuria). With tricuspid involvement the emboli are responsible for dyspnoea, cough, haemoptysis, and pleuritic chest pain. The annual risk of endocarditis for intravenous drug users is estimated at 2–5%. N.B. Recent guidelines suggest that only patients at the highest risk of infective endocarditis should be given prophylactic antibiotics prior to bacteraemia-producing procedures.

Warrell DA et al., *Oxford Textbook of Medicine*, Fifth Edition, Oxford University Press, 2010, Section 16.9.2, Infective endocarditis.

87. C. Mitral valve replacement

Indications for surgery in mitral stenosis, the diagnosis here, include: (1) significant symptoms limiting daily activities; (2) episode of acute pulmonary oedema with no obvious precipitant; (3) recurrent systemic emboli; (4) pulmonary oedema in pregnancy (consider emergency valvotomy); (5) deterioration due to AF that does not improve with medical treatment. Valve replacement is indicated if there is significant valvular calcification (as here), or the valve is severely diseased.

Ramrakha P, Hill J, *Oxford Handbook of Cardiology*, First Edition, Oxford University Press, 2006, Chapter 3, Valvular heart disease, Mitral stenosis guidelines.

88. A. Nitrates may relieve breathlessness

Breathlessness in mitral stenosis may be improved by the use of nitrates or diuretics. Beta-blockers may also be of value in reducing heart rate and improving exercise tolerance. Doppler is useful in determining the degree of mitral stenosis and hence the need for surgical intervention. Anticoagulation is not just recommended if there is thrombus in the left atrium, and may be considered if there is persistent atrial fibrillation or left atrial enlargement.

Ramrakha P, Hill J, *Oxford Handbook of Cardiology*, First Edition, Oxford University Press, 2006, Chapter 3, Valvular heart disease.

89. C. Erythromycin

This lady clearly has a history of sudden death at a young age in her family. This should alert you to the possibility of significant underlying familial cardiac disease. The development of torsades de pointes (twisting of the points/polymorphic ventricular tachycardia) is strongly linked with prolongation of the QT interval. There are two main familial causes of the long QT syndrome that you will need to know for the purposes of the exam. Jervell–Lange–Neilsen syndrome is inherited in an autosomal recessive pattern and is associated with congenital deafness. Romano–Ward syndrome is inherited in an autosomal dominant pattern and is not associated with deafness. Various medications are also implicated in prolongation of the QT interval including erythromycin.

It may well be that a combination of an underlying familial predisposition plus the culprit drug led to sufficient prolongation of the QT to cause torsades de pointes. The remaining drugs have no effect on the QT interval except magnesium. Magnesium is used as the emergency treatment for this condition but in intravenous form (usually 2 g magnesium sulphate).

Abrams DJ et al., Long QT syndrome, *British Medical Journal* 2010;340:b4815. http://www.bmj.com/content/340/bmj.b4815.full?ath_user=nhsdkelly006&ath_ttok=%3CTIAKpKPZl193MZoKug%3E.

90. D. Metoprolol

The initial priority is heart rate control and the safest, most effective medication in this situation is a beta-blocker. As this is the first documented episode of palpitations, it would seem reasonable to try and attain sinus rhythm in the longer term. Options include flecainide and amiodarone. Flecainide would be best avoided due to the previous history of significant IHD. If there were evidence of decompensation, the treatment is DC cardioversion.

Ramrakha P, Hill J, *Oxford Handbook of Cardiology*, First Edition, Oxford University Press, 2006, Chapter 10, Arrhythmias, Atrial fibrillation: management.

91. C. Prominent lower zone vasculature versus upper zone

Chest X-ray findings in congestive cardiac failure are loss of clearly defined vascular markings, thickened interlobular septa (Kerley B lines in the lung periphery), effusions (which can be unilateral), and multiple patchy air space opacities, and the heart is often enlarged. Vascular diversion occurs, with basal oligaemia, upper lobe hyperaemia.

Dahnert W, *Radiology Review Manual*, Fifth Edition, Lippincott Williams & Wilkins, 2003, Cardiovascular disorders, pp. 624–625.

92. E. Traditional angiography

This patient has chest pain which is not classical for angina, but his diabetes and smoking puts him into a higher risk group for CAD. Guidance from NICE recommends if the estimated risk is between 61% and 90% then angiography should be considered as the most important investigation. The NICE guidance tables put his level of risk at around 70%. The reason for progressing to angiography is because other investigations such as exercise testing do not categorically exclude coronary artery disease.

NICE guidelines: Chest pain of recent onset: assessment and diagnosis. https://www.nice.org.uk/guidance/cg95.

93. E. Verapamil

Limited evidence for angiographic intervention in post-cocaine myocardial infarction suggests that it is associated with an increased rate of haemorrhagic complications. As such, pharmacological intervention is usually attempted first. Beta-blockers exacerbate cocaine-induced vasoconstriction and are therefore contraindicated. Calcium channel blockers such as verapamil are the next agents of choice after GTN infusion. Only if patients fail to respond to calcium antagonists is coronary artery instrumentation usually considered. Benzodiazepines are also of value in managing acute anxiety associated with cocaine use.

Ramrakha P et al., *Oxford Handbook of Acute Medicine*, Third Edition, Oxford University Press, 2010.

94. D. Nitroprusside

This patient has acute mitral regurgitation, most probably due to rupture of the posteromedial papillary muscle. Anterior MI is less likely to cause mitral regurgitation, but when it does it occurs because of rupture of the anterolateral papillary muscle. Treatment with vasodilators such as sodium nitroprusside should be commenced as early as possible after haemodynamic monitoring is available. Crucial to prognosis is appropriate timing of surgical intervention with respect to repair of the valve.

Ramrakha P et al., *Oxford Handbook of Acute Medicine*, Third Edition, Oxford University Press, 2010.

http://ohacmed.oxfordmedicine.com/cgi/content/full/3/1/med-9780199230921-div1-01018.

95. B. Carvedilol in place of atenolol

Carvedilol in heart failure is associated with an improvement in life expectancy. It can in the initial stages, however, exacerbate symptoms of heart failure, so slow uptitration is recommended. Spironolactone is also shown to improve outcomes. Valsartan had an effect on heart failure hospitalizations. Loop diuretics, whilst improving symptoms, are not associated with improving prognosis. There is no evidence that amiodarone improves prognosis in this setting.

Longmore M et al., *Oxford Handbook of Clinical Medicine*, Eighth Edition, Oxford University Press, 2010, Chapter 3, Cardiovascular medicine, Heart failure—management.

96. E. Unstable angina

The signs, symptoms, ECG changes, and risk factors are typical of an acute coronary syndrome. The absence of troponin release excludes myocardial infarction according to its universal definition.

Wyatt JP et al., *Oxford Handbook of Emergency Medicine*, Fourth Edition, Oxford University Press, 2012.

97. C. Mesenteric angina

Most pathologies have already been excluded. The patient has a history of arteriosclerosis (peripheral vascular disease having already been demonstrated), and therefore mesenteric artery ischaemia is a possibility. His symptoms are characteristic. The long history of type I diabetes makes autonomic neuropathy possible but such individuals do not develop abdominal pain but rather delayed gastric emptying or nocturnal diarrhoea.

Warrell DA et al., *Oxford Textbook of Medicine*, Fifth Edition, Oxford University Press, 2010, Section 15.17, Vascular and collagen disorders.

98. A. Chest X-ray

The symptoms of acute onset chest pain radiating to the back, coupled with aortic regurgitation, raise the possibility of aortic dissection. Chest X-ray is abnormal in 90% of cases, with separation of intimal calcium and left-sided pleural effusion, both features seen in dissection. It is important not to wait for blood tests before arranging further imaging, as this may delay appropriate intervention. Given the history, this patient should absolutely not progress directly to thrombolysis.

Myerson SG et al., *Emergencies in Cardiology*, Second Edition, Oxford University Press, 2010, Chapter 11, Aortic dissection, Investigations.

99. B. 100 mmHg

In accelerated hypertension, an initial target for lowering of diastolic blood pressure is usually set at 100 mmHg, or 15–20 mmHg of reduction, whichever is greater. In patients with early changes, oral therapy may be appropriate, using beta-blockade or calcium channel blockers. In those with heart failure or very severe hypertension, parenteral therapy with labetalol or sodium nitroprusside is preferable. If renal function allows, then ACE inhibition should be considered as patients often have high circulating levels of renin.

Ramrakha P et al., *Oxford Handbook of Acute Medicine*, Third Edition, Oxford University Press, 2010.

100. D. Inter-dialysis ABPM

Arguments can be made for measuring both pre- and post-dialysis blood pressures for estimating control. In practice however it is ABPM measured during the period between dialyses which provides the best estimate of blood pressure control. Achieving blood pressure control of course is very difficult and patients often require multiple agents.

Levy J et al., *Oxford Handbook of Dialysis*, Third Edition, Oxford University Press, 2009, Chapter 11, Complications of ESKD: cardiovascular disease, BP control in patients on haemodialysis.

101. D. Nicorandil

GI ulceration, skin ulceration, and ulcers of the mucosal membranes have been reported. These tend to be refractory to treatment and most only respond to withdrawal of nicorandil treatment. Whilst metformin is associated with GI symptoms, these are abdominal bloating and diarrhoea, rather than ulceration. ACE inhibitors are associated with dry cough, and calcium channel antagonists with peripheral oedema.

Ramrakha P, Hill J, *Oxford Handbook of Cardiology*, Second Edition. Oxford University Press, 2012, Chapter 2, Drugs for the heart.

102. D. Ventricular fibrillation

This man has suffered an out-of-hospital cardiac arrest against a background of likely ischaemic heart disease. The most likely cause is an acute myocardial infarction complicated by a fatal arrhythmia. Aortic dissection is said to present more commonly with a tearing pain radiating to the back. Acute mitral regurgitation, VSD and left ventricular wall rupture are usually seen later, post-myocardial infarction (approximately 48 hours or more later). These three conditions tend not to be associated with sudden death but would present with fulminant left ventricular failure/cardiogenic shock as opposed to sudden cardiac death.

Banerjee A, Hargreaves C, *Oxford Specialist Handbook: A Resuscitation Room Guide*, Oxford University Press, 2007, Chapter 4, Coronary artery disease.

103. D. Indapamide

In Afro-Caribbeans or patients >55 years of age, a calcium channel antagonist is the initial therapy of choice. In patients who do not tolerate this a thiazide-like diuretic, not a thiazide itself, is recommended. As such, chlortalidone or indapamide are the second line agents of choice and are preferred to bendroflumethiazide or hydrochlorthiazide in the new NICE hypertension guidelines issued in 2011. In those under 55 years and of Caucasian origin, an ACE inhibitor is the initial therapy of choice.

NICE guidelines: Hypertension in adults: diagnosis and management. http://publications.nice.org.uk/hypertension-cg127.

104. B. Glyceryl trinitrate

Cocaine use is associated with vasoconstriction, which in turn drives myocardial ischaemia. This can be significantly worsened by beta-blockade; therefore, in this situation nitrates (e.g. GTN infusion) and calcium channel antagonists are the treatment of choice. Anti-platelet therapy with aspirin, clopidogrel, and a therapy with a factor X inhibitor such as fondaparinux are also likely to be of value, but will impact less on his chest pain than relieving vasospasm.

Ramrakha P, Hill J, *Oxford Handbook of Cardiology*, Second Edition, Oxford University Press, 2012, Chapter 5, Interventional cardiology.

105. D. Periprocedural myocardial infarction is a marker of atherosclerotic burden rather than an indicator of patient prognosis

Periprocedural myocardial infarction is classified separately from spontaneous myocardial infarction. The incidence of periprocedural myocardial infarction is between 5–30%. It is defined as a rise in either troponin T or troponin I of at least five times the upper limit of normal 8–12 hours after the procedure. Spontaneous myocardial infarction is defined as a troponin rise of at least three times the upper limit of normal. Only patients who complain of chest pain and/or who have ECG evidence of ischaemia after PCI should be screened for periprocedural myocardial infarction. If all patients were screened, it is likely there would be many false positive cases identified. In general, periprocedural myocardial infarction does not affect patient prognosis but rather is a marker of atherosclerotic burden and case complexity. Complex lesions and complex procedures increase the risk of periprocedural myocardial infarction. Increasing age is a risk factor for periprocedural myocardial infarction. Other risk factors include diabetes mellitus, chronic kidney disease, LV dysfunction and multi vessel disease.

Prasad A, Herrmann J, Myocardial infarction due to percutaneous coronary intervention, *New England Journal of Medicine* 2011;364:453–464.

106. A. Left anterior descending in-stent restenosis

In-stent restenosis is said to occur in around 10% of those who undergo coronary angioplasty with stent deployment, although it occurs more commonly in patients with type 2 diabetes. Given the ECG changes are seen in the anterolateral leads, the likely territory is the left anterior descending artery. It is extremely rare to have acute stent thrombosis five years after angioplasty, and if it did occur, would result in ST-segment elevation on the ECG as opposed to ST-segment deviation seen here. Coronary vasospasm also tends to cause ST-segment elevation rather than depression.

Ramrakha P, Hill J, *Oxford Handbook of Cardiology*, Second Edition, Oxford University Press, 2012, Chapter 6, Heart failure.

107. B. COPD with decreased FEV1

There are a number of contraindications to cardiac transplant, which include severe concomitant disease affecting another organ system, of which COPD is a clear example. The range of contraindications are listed: (1) age greater than 65 years; (2) severe pulmonary hypertension; (3) recent (past 6–8 weeks) history of pulmonary infarction; (4) evidence of significant end-organ damage due to diabetes; (5) any chronic illness affecting survival or function status; (6) symptomatic or severe peripheral vascular and carotid disease; (7) active infection; (8) severe, chronic, or irreversible functional damage to any vital organ (including renal, pulmonary, hepatic failure); (9) severe obesity (greater than 130% ideal body weight) or cachexia (less than 80% ideal body weight); (10) drug, alcohol, or tobacco abuse in the previous six months; (11) psychiatric illness or poor medical compliance; (12) sctive or recent malignancy; (13) HIV infection.

Ramrakha P, Hill J, *Oxford Handbook of Cardiology*, Second Edition, Oxford University Press, 2012, Chapter 7, Heart muscle diseases.

108. B. Switch his spironolactone for eplerenone

After the results of the RALES study, spironolactone became the default aldosterone antagonist for the treatment of heart failure, although it is associated with gynaecomastia. The main body of evidence to support the use of eplerenone is in the post MI population, although it is also used in cases where spironolactone is not tolerated, particularly as it is not associated with gynaecomastia. Given that the patient has stable symptoms of heart failure, a straight switch between the two agents is therefore the most appropriate option. Chronic use of loop diuretics is not associated with improved outcomes. Whilst ACE inhibitor and ARB combination therapy do improve symptoms of heart failure, they are not as effective as the combination of ACE inhibitor and aldosterone antagonist therapy.

Ramrakha P, Hill J, *Oxford Handbook of Cardiology*, Second Edition, Oxford University Press, 2012, Chapter 7, Heart muscle diseases.

109. E. Ventricular septal defect

Acute VSD is seen approximately 24 hours after MI, anterior infarction is associated with apical VSD, inferior infarction is associated with basal VSD. Symptoms are those of cardiogenic shock seen here, coupled with a harsh pansystolic murmur. In this case with significant hypotension, early intra-aortic balloon pump and surgery are important management options, although operative mortality is very high. Acute MR is more usually associated with inferior MI, and ventricular free wall rupture leads to sudden death in two-thirds of those who suffer it.

Ramrakha P, Hill J, *Oxford Handbook of Cardiology*, Second Edition, Oxford University Press, 2012, Chapter 5, Interventional cardiology.

110. D. Bisoprolol

Beta-blockade is the next most appropriate intervention in patients with heart failure due to left ventricular dysfunction who appear to be in approximate fluid balance. A cardioselective beta-blocker such as bisoprolol or carvedilol is most appropriate. In cases of fluid overload, management with diuretics followed by introduction of a beta-blocker would be the best option. Biventricular pacing is reserved for patients with symptoms despite maximal therapy.

NICE guidelines: Chronic heart failure: quick reference guide. http://www.nice.org.uk/guidance/CG108/QuickRefGuide/pdf/English.

111. D. Ivabradine

Ivabradine is a pure heart rate lowering agent, acting by selective and specific inhibition of the cardiac pacemaker I(f) current that controls the spontaneous diastolic depolarization in the sinus node and regulates heart rate. The cardiac effects are specific to the sinus node with no effect on intra-atrial, atrioventricular or intraventricular conduction times, nor on myocardial contractility, or ventricular repolarization. The SHIFT study in patients with heart failure and resting heart rate >70 demonstrated a clinically and statistically significant relative risk reduction of 18% in the rate of the primary composite endpoint of cardiovascular mortality and hospitalisation for worsening heart failure (hazard ratio: 0.82, 95% CI [0.75;0.90]—p<0.0001) apparent within three months of initiation of treatment. The other options are all calcium channel antagonists which have not been shown to impact on outcomes.

Ivabradine: summary of product characteristics. http://www.medicines.org.uk/emc/medicine/17188/SPC/#INDICATIONS.

112. E. Fondaparinux

NICE guidelines on acute coronary syndrome management suggest that fondaparinux should be added to dual anti-platelet therapy as long as the patient does not have a high risk of bleeding, and angiography is not planned within a 24-hour period. If angiography is planned within 24 hours then unfractionated heparin is probably a better option. GP2b3a inhibitors are considered for patients thought to have a >3% risk of a coronary event within a six-month period according to GRACE registry criteria.

NICE guidelines: Unstable angina and NSTEMI. https://www.nice.org.uk/guidance/CG94.

113. D. Ivabradine

Ivabradine is indicated in chronic heart failure NYHA II to IV class with systolic dysfunction, in patients in sinus rhythm and whose heart rate is >70 bpm at rest, in combination with standard therapy including beta-blocker therapy or when beta-blocker therapy is contraindicated or not tolerated. The recommendation to initiate ivabradine is based on the SHIFT study, which was a large multicentre, international, randomized double-blind placebo controlled outcome trial conducted in 6505 adult patients with stable chronic CHF , NYHA class II to IV, with a reduced left ventricular ejection fraction (LVEF <35%) and a resting heart rate >70 bpm. Patients received standard care including beta-blockers (89%), ACE inhibitors and/or angiotensin II antagonists (91%), diuretics (83%), and anti-aldosterone agents (60%). In the ivabradine group, 67% of patients were treated with 7.5 mg twice a day. The median follow-up duration was 22.9 months. Treatment with ivabradine was associated with an average reduction in heart rate of 15 bpm from a baseline value of 80 bpm. The difference in heart rate between ivabradine and placebo arms was 10.8 bpm at 28 days, 9.1 bpm at 12 months and 8.3 bpm at 24 months. The study demonstrated a clinically and statistically significant relative risk reduction of 18% in the rate of the primary composite endpoint of cardiovascular mortality and hospitalization for worsening heart failure (hazard ratio: 0.82, 95%CI [0.75;0.90]—p<0.0001) apparent within three months of initiation of treatment. The absolute risk reduction was 4.2%.

Ivabradine prescribing information. http://www.medicines.org.uk/emc/medicine/17188/SPC/.

114. B. Monophasic R in V1

The Brugada criteria may be helpful in differentiating VT from SVT. They are listed here (a monophasic R in V1 favours ventricular tachycardia):

Broad complexes + rbbb-like qrs pattern on 12 lead ECG:

Lead V1:
- Monophasic r or qr or rs favours VT
- Triphasic rsr favours SVT

Lead V6:
- r to s ratio <1 (r wave < s wave) favours VT
- qs or qr favours VT
- Monophasic r favours VT
- Triphasic favours SVT
- r to s ratio >1 (r wave > s wave) favours SVT

Broad complexes + lbbb-like qrs on 12 lead ECG:

Lead V1 or V2:

Any of these:
- r >30 msec
- >60 msec to nadir s
- Notched s favours VT

Lead V6:
- Presence of any q wave, qr or qs favours VT
- No q wave in lead V6 favours SVT.

Adapted from *Circulation*, 83, 5, P Brugada, J Brugada, I Mont et al., `A new approach to the differential diagnosis of a regular tachycardia with a wide QRS complex'. Copyright (1991) with permission from Wolters Kluwer Health, Inc.

Longmore M et al., *Oxford Handbook of Clinical Medicine*, Eighth Edition, Oxford University Press, 2010.

115. B. Digoxin

In this situation, successful cardioversion to sinus rhythm is very unlikely. Flecanide is contraindicated anyway in this situation because of the previous history of ischaemic heart disease, and amiodarone in this case would need to be delivered intravenously via a large bore central line. Out of the options for rate control, both diltiazem and bisoprolol may further reduce blood pressure and also worsen the heart failure; therefore digoxin, which will control rate and is positively inotropic (i.e. improve cardiac function) is the most appropriate choice.

Ramrakha P, Hill J, *Oxford Handbook of Cardiology*, Second Edition, Oxford University Press, 2012, Chapter 10, Invasive electrocardiography.

116. A. intravenous diamorphine

In this situation, where blood pressure is relatively preserved, saturations have improved a little, but the patient is very distressed with an elevated respiratory rate, diamorphine is a reasonable option. It serves to relieve anxiety, act as a vasodilator, and reduce sympathetic drive. Inotropes are likely to worsen myocardial ischaemia and should therefore be avoided if possible. Ventilation is reserved for patients who fail to respond to medical therapy.

Morrell Nicholas W, Firth John D, *Pulmonary oedema—Oxford Textbook of Medicine*, Fifth Edition, Oxford University Press, 2010, Chapter 16, Cardiovascular disorders.

1. **A 68-year-old man who is already treated with ramipril post anterior myocardial infarction comes to the clinic for review with worsening symptoms of cardiac failure. You elect to treat him with furosemide. Which of the following fits correctly with the mode of action of furosemide?**

   A. Inhibits action of carbonic anhydrase in the proximal convoluted tubule

   B. Inhibits the co-transport of $Na^+/K^+/2Cl^-$ in the thick ascending limb of the loop of Henlé

   C. Inhibits NaCl transport in the distal convoluted tubule

   D. Blocks sodium channels in the collecting tubules

   E. Promotes osmotic diuresis

2. **A 69-year-old woman is reviewed in clinic. She has a history of recurrent ventricular tachycardia and has been treated with long-term amiodarone therapy having refused electrophysiological investigation and an implantable cardioverter defibrillator. She noticed a swelling in her neck about four months earlier. On examination she feels warm and has a fine tremor. Her pulse is regular at 95 bpm and her BP is 143/95 mmHg. She has a palpable goitre and her thyroid gland is mildly tender. Investigations: thyroid-stimulating hormone <0.4 mU/l (0.4–5.0), anti-thyroid peroxidase antibodies 240 IU/ml (<50). Which of the following is the most appropriate treatment?**

   A. Carbimazole

   B. Carbimazole and thyroxine (block replace regimen)

   C. NSAIDs

   D. Prednisolone

   E. Surgery

3. **A 52-year-old alcoholic man is found by his friend unconscious next to an empty bottle of whisky and an empty bottle of temazepam 10 mg. The friend calls an ambulance and when he is brought to the emergency department the man is deeply unconscious. On examination his respiratory rate is 8, his BP is 90/50, and his pupils are dilated and poorly reactive. Investigations (arterial blood gas): PaO_2 8.2, $PaCO_2$ 7.5, pH 7.2. Which of the following is the most appropriate next step?**
   A. Flumazenil
   B. Naloxone
   C. Intubation and ventilation
   D. Oropharyngeal airway
   E. Commence regular neurological observations (every 10 minutes)

4. **Alkylating agents are a group of cytotoxic drugs that exert their biological activities via which of the following mechanisms?**
   A. DNA crosslinking
   B. Antimicrotubule activity
   C. Folic acid antagonist
   D. Pyrimidine analogue
   E. Purine analogue

5. **You are investigating small molecule kinase inhibitors for the treatment of solid tumours. You are aware that different molecules target different tumour growth factor receptors and their function. Which of the following targets does pazopanib act on? Options**
   A. VEGFR, PDGFR, and c-kit
   B. HER-1 and HER-2
   C. bcr-abl
   D. EDGFR and c-kit
   E. HER-1, HER-2, and c-kit

6. **An 18-year-old woman with a long history of deliberate self harm attends the A&E department telling you she has ingested up to 20 ml of paraquat-based weed killer some 30 minutes earlier. On examination her BP is 110/70, her pulse is 80 and regular, and she complains of a burning sensation in her mouth and throat. Which of the following is the most appropriate initial management?**
    A. Activated charcoal
    B. Gastric lavage
    C. Omeprazole
    D. Haemofiltration
    E. Gaviscon

7. **A 42-year-old woman with advanced breast cancer and a prognosis of only 2–3 months comes to the clinic with intractable pain going down her right leg. She has constant pain in her right posterior thigh and calf, radiating down to her big toe. She is taking BD MST at a dose of 100 mg BD, and regular paracetamol. Her creatinine is elevated at 220 µmol/l. An MRI scan shows invasion of the right foramen of S1. Which of the following is the most appropriate next step?**
    A. Add diclofenac 50 mg BD
    B. Increase her MST
    C. Switch to s/c diamorphine
    D. TENS machine
    E. Arrange an S1 spinal block

8. **A 46-year-old man presents with nausea, polyuria, and polydypsia. He has been seeing his GP over the past few months for increasing shortness of breath and has been prescribed a salbutamol and steroid inhaler. On examination he has a BP of 155/82, his pulse is 80 and regular. There are sparse crackles on auscultation of the chest. You notice some raised red nodules on both shins. Investigations: Hb 12.9, WCC 8.0, PLT 202, Na 137, K 4.0, Cr 132, Ca 2.93. Which of the following treatments is likely to be most effective in reducing his calcium?**
    A. Risedronate
    B. Furosemide
    C. Bendroflumethiazide
    D. Prednisolone 40 mg
    E. Prednisolone 5 mg

9. **Fomepizole (4-methylpyrazole) is indicated for use as an antidote in confirmed or suspected anti-freeze poisoning. Its mechanism of action is:**

   A. HMG-CoA reductase inhibitor

   B. Xanthine oxidase inhibitor

   C. Alcohol dehydrogenase inhibitor

   D. Cyclo-oxygenase inhibitor

   E. Na^+/K^+ ATPase pump inhibitor

10. **A 43-year-old woman comes to the clinic a few months after receiving a liver transplant. She is receiving a potent immunosuppressive regime with mycophenolate, ciclosporin, and prednisolone. She complains of severe diarrhoea which she originally thought was due to a gastrointestinal infection. Her bowels are open some 8–12 times per day with non-bloody diarrhoea and mucus. She has a postural drop and mildly tender abdomen on palpation. Investigations: Hb 11.9 g/dl (11.5–16.5), WCC 9.2 x 10^9/l (4–11), PLT 191 x 10^9/l (130–400), Na 137 mmol/l (135–145), K 4.3 mmol/l (3.5–5.0), Cr 132 micromol/l (50–90). Which of the following is the most likely cause of her diarrhoea?**

    A. Cryptosporidium

    B. Ciclosporin

    C. New onset ulcerative colitis

    D. Collagenous colitis

    E. Mycophenolate

11. **A known epileptic has had a number of convulsions with incomplete recovery over the preceding 35 minutes; these have been witnessed by her mother who also informs you that she usually takes carbamazepine to control her seizures. Which of the following statements is correct?**

    A. This is status epilepticus

    B. She should be given IV midazolam

    C. In the acute setting it is important to test her blood glucose level, electrolytes, and carbamazepine levels

    D. Thiopentone is the second-line treatment

    E. If the seizures settle she needs no further investigation

12. **You are evaluating immunosuppression protocols for patients undergoing liver transplantation. Potential options include sirolimus, tacrolimus, azathioprine, and ciclosporin. Which of the following agents is known to inhibit mTOR?**
    A. Tacrolimus
    B. Sirolimus
    C. Azathioprine
    D. Ciclosporin
    E. Prednisolone

13. **A 34-year-old man, who has had a previous renal transplant and takes ciclosporin, goes to see the duty doctor with oropharyngeal candidiasis. He is prescribed a course of ketoconazole. Other medication of note includes ramipril and indapamide for control of blood pressure. On his return to the renal clinic a short time later his BP is 132/82, pulse is 72 and regular. His creatinine has deteriorated from 145 µmol/l to 235 µmol/l. Which of the following is the most likely diagnosis?**
    A. Ciclosporin toxicity
    B. Hypertensive renal disease
    C. Ketoconazole-related nephritis
    D. Chronic rejection
    E. Ramipril toxicity

14. **You start a 40-year-old woman on oral steroid treatment for her severe asthma. You should warn her about the potential side effects, but which one of the following is not a recognized side effect of steroid treatment?**
    A. Hypoglycaemia
    B. Increased blood pressure
    C. Osteoporosis
    D. Increased risk of peptic ulcer disease
    E. Mood change

15. You plan to start a patient on azathioprine for inflammatory bowel disease, which was recently confirmed following multiple colonic biopsies. Which test would be most useful to carry out first?

A. Thiopurine methyltransferase (TPMT) levels
B. Catechol-O-methyltransferase (COMT) levels
C. Anti-tissue tranglutaminase (tTG) antibody levels
D. HLA B27 testing
E. Faecal calprotectin testing

16. A 23-year-old man comes to the sexually transmitted diseases clinic because he has developed a painless ulcer on his penis some two weeks after returning from a holiday to Spain with his friends. He admits to unprotected sex on a number of occasions during the holiday. Dark field microscopy of fluid from the ulcer suggests a diagnosis of primary syphilis. Which of the following is the most appropriate treatment (he is penicillin allergic)?

A. Doxycycline for 14 days
B. Azithromycin single dose
C. Ciprofloxacin for 14 days
D. Clindamycin for 7 days
E. Cephalexin for 7 days

17. A 28-year-old woman comes to the clinic requesting advice about vaccination as she is planning to join her partner on a trip abroad. She is three months pregnant. When thinking about destinations, which of the following vaccination requirements is contraindicated in pregnancy?

A. Tetanus
B. Yellow fever
C. Hepatitis A
D. Diptheria
E. Hepatitis B

18. **From the list of medications below, which would be the most appropriate first-line antiepileptic medication for generalized epilepsy?**
    A. Sodium valproate
    B. Carbamazepine
    C. Topiramate
    D. Levetiracetam
    E. Ethosuximide

19. **From the list below what would be the the first-line antiepileptic of choice for focal seizures?**
    A. Phenytoin
    B. Carbamazepine
    C. Topiramate
    D. Levetiracetam
    E. Ethosuximide

20. **Which one of the following diseases is intravenous immunoglobulin not a treatment option for?**
    A. Guillain–Barré syndrome
    B. Myasthenia gravis
    C. Multifocal motor neuropathy
    D. Limbic encephalitis
    E. Goodpasture's disease with neurological complications

21. **A 33-year-old woman is seen in the chest clinic. She has a salbutamol inhaler 100 mcg PRN and beclomethasone dipropionate inhaler 400 mcg bd. She still suffers from asthma exacerbations. She reports that her GP prescribed her an oral course of steroids a couple of weeks ago for her asthma exacerbation. She has never had an intensive care unit or high dependency unit admission for her asthma. What would be your next step to manage her asthma?**
    A. Add a long-acting beta2 agonist inhaler (salmeterol)
    B. Add a leukotriene receptor antagonist (montelukast)
    C. Add a long-acting muscarinic receptor antagonist (tiotropium)
    D. Increase the beclomethasone to 800 mcg bd
    E. Keep on a low-dose prednisolone tablet od

22. **A 56-year-old man with a history of ischaemic heart disease comes to the clinic complaining of painful defecation. His GP was concerned about ischaemic colitis, but on examination you found evidence of anal fissuring and ulceration. Which of the following medications is most likely to have contributed to his presentation?**
    A. Amlodipine
    B. Indapamide
    C. Isosorbide mononitrate
    D. Nicorandil
    E. Ramipril

23. **You are reviewing situations in which osteonecrosis of the jaw may occur and doing a literature review. Which of the following medications is known to be most associated with osteonecrosis of the jaw?**
    A. Non-steroidal anti-inflammatory agents
    B. Sunitinib
    C. ACE inhibitors
    D. Calcium and vitamin D
    E. Cinacalet

24. **A 42-year-old man is admitted with smoke inhalation after a fire at the polyurethane foam factory where he works. He is complaining of dizziness and chest tightness, is unable to stand due to weakness, and seems confused. On examination his BP is 100/50, his pulse is 92 and regular. There are bilateral crackles on auscultation of the chest. You administer 100% O_2 via mask. Which of the following additional therapies is most appropriate?**
    A. Methylene blue
    B. Vitamin C
    C. Hydroxycobalamin
    D. Bisoprolol
    E. Diazepam

25. **A 67-year-old woman with long-standing Parkinson's comes to the neurology clinic for review. She is taking a large dose of levodopa but is suffering from increasing on/off phenomena so that she is frozen for large periods of the day. She is also taking ramipril and amlodipine. Which of the following is likely to be most helpful with respect to on/off phenomena?**
   A. Entacapone
   B. Apomorphine
   C. Amitriptyline
   D. Selegiline
   E. Pergolide

26. **A 62-year-old woman is admitted unconscious having been found by her home help with an empty bottle of amitriptyline at her side. She has recently lost her husband due to cancer. On examination she had a Glasgow coma score of 5 with sluggish dilated pupils. Her pulse was regular at 100 bpm and her blood pressure was 95/50 mmHg. Investigations: ECG: sinus rhythm at 100 bpm with non-sustained ventricular tachycardia, QRS duration 140 ms (80–120 ms); blood gases: pH 7.15. Which of the following is the most appropriate treatment to reduce the risks of sustained VT?**
   A. Lignocaine
   B. Bicarbonate
   C. Amiodarone
   D. Quinidine
   E. Phenytoin

27. **A 58-year-old woman, on treatment for refractory hypertension with felodipine, bendroflumethiazide, doxazosin, perindopril, and irbesartan, is found on routine screening to have a corrected serum calcium of 2.8 mmol/l. She is otherwise in good health. Her chest X-ray is normal. There is no paraproteinaemia on electrophoresis and her parathormone level is 2.1 pmol/l. What is the cause of her hypercalcaemia?**
   A. Calcium channel blocker
   B. Diuretic
   C. Angiotensin II receptor blocker
   D. Alpha-blocker
   E. ACE inhibitor

28. **A 47-year-old man underwent a hypophysectomy for an adenoma causing bitemporal hemianopia and is started on the following therapy—levothyroxine 200 mcg daily, desmopressin spray 10 mcg bd, hydrocortisone 20 mg morning and 10 mg evening, fludrocortisone 100 mcg daily, and testosterone 40 mg daily. Which of the drugs is inappropriately prescribed?**

    A. Desmopressin
    B. Fludrocortisone
    C. Hydrocortisone
    D. Levothyroxine
    E. Testosterone

29. **A 43-year-old woman is admitted with severe community-acquired pneumonia. Her background is notable only for severe psoriasis and psoriatic arthritis, for which she takes methotrexate 20 mg weekly. She also takes folic acid 5 mg weekly and co-codamol 30/500 as required. Initial blood results show haemoglobin 10.2 g/dl, total white cell count 2.3 x10^9/litre, neutrophils 0.9 x 10^9/litre, platelets 88 x 10^9/litre. She is commenced on intravenous fluids and antibiotics. Her methotrexate is due the following day. Regarding her psoriasis and psoriatic arthritis treatment, select the most appropriate management.**

    A. Continue methotrexate and change folic acid to folinic acid
    B. Continue methotrexate and folic acid
    C. Reduce methotrexate to 10 mg per week and increase folic acid to 5 mg daily
    D. Withhold methotrexate and give folinic acid
    E. Withhold methotrexate and increase folic acid to 5 mg daily

30. **A 52-year-old woman is admitted after deliberate ingestion of arsenic. What is the antidote of choice?**

    A. 2,3-dimercaptopropanesulphonate (DMPS)
    B. Dicobalt edetate
    C. Desferrioxamine
    D. Pralidoxime
    E. Atropine

31. **An 88-year-old man is admitted with decreased mobility and dysuria. Four days earlier he had a nephrostomy tube inserted because he had left ureteric obstruction due to a stone. He was awaiting ureteroscopy and stone extraction. He had a non-ST elevation myocardial infarction (NSTEMI) one year earlier and also suffered from osteoarthritis in both hips and knees, osteomalacia due to secondary hyperparathyroidism, pleural plaques from asbestos exposure, hiatus hernia, and chronic renal impairment. He has also had two episodes of coliform septicaemia in the previous six months. He is taking ciprofloxacin, paracetamol, oxybutynin, bisoprolol, simvastatin, nicorandil, furosemide, alfacalcidol, lansoprazole, and calcichew D3. On examination he was dehydrated. Cognition was normal. Pulse was 65 bpm, sinus rhythm, and blood pressure was 122/70 mmHg. There was reduced air entry at the left lung base on auscultating the chest. A nephrostomy tube was in situ. His urine dipstick was +ve for blood, protein, leucocytes, and nitrites. Other blood results on admission were: Hb 11.2 g/dl (13–18), WBC 17.8 x 10^9/l (4–11), platelets 219 x 10^9/l (150–400), Na 136 mmol/l (137–144), K 4.9 mmol/l (3.5–4.9), HCO_3 17 mmol/l (19–24), creatinine 307 micromol/l (60–110) (166 two months ago), CRP 99 mg/l (<10), CK 155 U/l (24–195). He was rehydrated with intravenous fluids and, after discussion with the microbiologist, given intravenous vancomycin and coamoxiclav along with oral fluconazole. Renal ultrasound showed mild left hydronephrosis, and slight loss of cortical thickness in the right kidney. Two days later his creatinine was 575 and creatine kinase (CK) 2700. Which combination of drugs is most likely to explain these changes in CK and creatinine?**

    A. Alfacalcidol and vancomycin
    B. Ciprofloxacin and fluconazole
    C. Fluconazole and simvastatin
    D. Simvastatin and vancomycin
    E. Vancomycin and ciprofloxacin

32. **Which of the following may cause optic neuritis?**

    A. Rifampicin
    B. Isoniazid
    C. Ethambutol
    D. Streptomycin
    E. Pyrazinamide

33. **Which of the following is a direct factor Xa inhibitor?**

A. Rivaroxaban

B. Enoxaparin

C. Dabigatran

D. Unfractionated heparin

E. Clopidogrel

34. **A 42-year-old woman is given sevoflurane as part of general anaesthesia. This rapidly precipitates hyperthermia, rhabdomyolysis, and muscle rigidity. Which gene is most commonly mutated to cause this disorder?**

A. *RYR1*

B. *CFTR*

C. *FBN1*

D. *DMPK*

E. *SCN4A*

35. **You are asked to review a 25-year-old man who has been admitted under the psychiatrists with an acute psychotic episode thought to be related to schizophrenia. He has been managed with haloperidol, but you are asked to see him because he has developed a fever of 39°C, muscular rigidity, and difficulty swallowing. He is also complaining of pain and spasm affecting his neck. Which of the following is the most appropriate treatment for him?**

A. Diazepam

B. Bromocriptine

C. Dantrolene

D. Paracetamol

E. Levodopa

36. **A 55-year-old man is diagnosed with chronic phase CML requiring treatment. Which is the most appropriate therapy?**

A. Gemtuzumab

B. Imatinib

C. Rituximab

D. Cetuximab

E. Sunitinib

37. You are looking after an 80-year-old man with advanced prostate cancer, who is having problems with bone pain. Three days ago, he was started on 1 g paracetamol four times daily, but he does not think this helped much. He rates this pain 3/10. He has no known allergies. What do you think the next step should be in managing his pain?

    A. Stop paracetamol and start codeine
    B. Stop paracetamol and start morphine
    C. Continue paracetamol and encourage physiotherapy
    D. Start a syringe driver with morphine
    E. Continue paracetamol and add codeine

38. A 67-year-old man attends for a stress myocardial perfusion imaging. His past medical history includes hypertension, a transient ischaemic attack, severe psoriatic arthritis, and a recent productive cough. His current medication includes azathiorpine, clarithromycin, dipyridamole, lisinopril, and methotrexate. Which of these drugs is a contraindication to adenosine?

    A. Azathioprine
    B. Clarithromycin
    C. Dipyridamole
    D. Lisinopril
    E. Methotrexate

39. You are treating someone with a chemotherapy agent that has a high risk of causing tumour lysis syndrome. You give them allopurinol beforehand to prevent renal damage. What is the mechanism of action of this drug?

    A. HMG co-A reductase inhibitor
    B. Xanthine oxidase inhibitor
    C. Suppression of T cells
    D. Suppression of B cells
    E. Uricosuric

40. A 61-year-old man with multiple medical problems comes to the clinic complaining that the paracetamol he takes regularly for his osteoarthritis is no longer proving sufficient. You suspect that this may be due to a drug interaction. Which of the following medications is most likely to be responsible?
    A. Omeprazole
    B. Atenolol
    C. Metaclopramide
    D. Amoxicillin
    E. Metformin

41. A 62-year-old woman comes to the rheumatology clinic for review. She has suffered from rheumatoid arthritis for the past 10 years, and still has active synovitis despite methotrexate therapy. You decide to commence adalimumab. Which of the following correctly describes the mode of action of adalimumab?
    A. IL-1 receptor antagonist
    B. TNF antagonist
    C. TNF receptor antagonist
    D. IL-6 receptor antagonist
    E. IL-10 receptor antagonist

42. A 42-year-old man presents to the dermatology clinic with severe psoriasis. He has been taking ciclosporin and has completed a course of PUVA, but still has a significant PASI score of 22 and feels very depressed about his skin condition. Which of the following is the most appropriate next step?
    A. Oral prednisolone.
    B. Topical triamcinalone.
    C. Infliximab.
    D. Methotrexate.
    E. Cyclophosphamide.

43. **You are reviewing prescription of antibiotics in the local hospital and want to ensure that only antihistamine anti-emetics are prescribed for certain populations, particularly young women, because of the risk of acute dystonic reactions, and ensuring costs are kept to a minimum by not using more expensive agents. Which of the following is an antihistamine anti-emetic?**

    A. Metaclopramide
    B. Domperidone
    C. Prochlorperazine
    D. Hyoscine
    E. Cyclizine

44. **You are reviewing a 23-year-old patient with type 1 diabetes who has purchased an insulin pump so that she can transfer to pump therapy prior to trying to get pregnant. She is already relatively well controlled with a recent HbA1c measured at 7.5% (59 mmol/mol), but wants to minimize any weight gain and glycaemic excursions. Which of the following is the most appropriate insulin to put into her pump?**

    A. Insulin aspart
    B. Human mixtard 50:50
    C. Insulin glargine
    D. Insulin detemir
    E. NPH insulin

45. **Which is a typical side effect of olanzapine?**

    A. Akathisia
    B. Hypoadrenalism
    C. Hypoglycaemia
    D. Macroglossia
    E. Stevens–Johnson syndrome

46. **A 66-year-old woman is seen in clinic for review of type 2 diabetes. She has a past history of microalbuminuria, but is otherwise relatively free of diabetic complications. Medication includes a combination of pioglitazone 45 mg and metformin 1 g BD. On examination her BMI is 32 with increased abdominal adipose tissue, blood pressure is 155/80 mmHg, and she has bilateral pitting ankle oedema. Her recent bone mineral density has been within the normal range with a T score of −0.5. Which of the following is a recognized side effect of glitazone therapy?**

    A. Decreased peripheral fat
    B. Hypertension
    C. Increased central fat
    D. Increased bone mineral density
    E. Peripheral oedema without heart failure

47. **A 24-year-old woman who has manic depressive psychosis is found collapsed in a night club. She is known to be taking long-term atypical anti-psychotic therapy. She was out celebrating a hen night and it is unclear as to whether she took any illicit drugs. On examination she is hypertensive at 156/96. Her pulse is 95 and regular. She has a temperature of 39°C., has dilated pupils, and increased tone bilaterally. Investigations: Hb 12.3 g/dl, WCC 12.6 x 10⁹/l, PLT 203 x 10⁹/l, Na 133 mmol/l, K 5.7 mmol/l, creatinine 131 μmol/l, bicarbonate 17 mmol/l, PaO₂ 10.9 kPa, PaCO₂ 4.7 kPa, creatine kinase 784 U/l. Which of the following is the most likely diagnosis?**

    A. Ecstasy overdose
    B. Tardive dyskinesia
    C. Neuroleptic malignant syndrome
    D. Water intoxication
    E. LSD overdose

48. **A 63-year-old woman with type 2 diabetes was found to have a serum triglyceride concentration of 12 mmol/l. As part of her risk factor modification regimen, she was started on fenofibrate. Which of the following best describes the mode of action of fenofibrate?**

    A. Down-regulation of lipoprotein lipase
    B. HMG-CoA reductase inhibitor
    C. PPAR-alpha agonist

D. PPAR-delta agonist

E. PPAR-gamma agonist

49. **You are examining the range of 5HT agonists and antagonists and their indications. What is the role of the 5HT-2B receptor antagonist, sarpogrelate?**

A. Atypical anti-psychotic

B. Anti-platelet agent

C. Anti-emetic

D. Migraine therapy

E. Sedative

50. **A 51-year-old man is reviewed six weeks after an anterior myocardial infarction. His past medical history includes liver transplantation four years earlier. His medication comprises immunosuppressants including tacrolimus. He has developed impaired glucose tolerance and dyslipidaemia, with an HDL of 0.8 mmol/l and an LDL of 5.9 mmol/l. Which agent is most appropriate to improve his dyslipidaemia?**

A. Atorvastatin

B. Ezetimibe

C. Fenofibrate

D. Pravastatin

E. Simvastatin

51. **A 67-year-old man is admitted to hospital because of angina. He smokes 20 cigarettes per day and has a history of chronic obstructive pulmonary disease. His medication includes aspirin, diltiazem, isosorbide mononitrate, nicorandil, ramipril, and simvastatin. He has proven to be intolerant of beta-blockers. You recommend ivabradine as an additional anti-anginal agent. Which of the following side effects should you warn him of?**

A. Heart block

B. Hypertension

C. Luminosities within the visual fields

D. Postural hypotension

E. Tachycardia

52. **A 71-year-old woman is unable to take risedronate therapy due to problems with severe oesophagitis. Instead she is prescribed six-monthly denosumab SC injections. When is the nadir of carboxy-terminal collagen crosslinks reduction reached in response to denosumab therapy?**

    A. Three days
    B. Two weeks
    C. Four weeks
    D. Two months
    E. Four months

53. **A 74-year-old woman is treated with strontium ranelate therapy for her osteoporosis as she is unable to tolerate bisphosphonate therapy. She is concerned about the side effect profile and asks you a number of questions about this. Which of the following represents a commonly reported adverse event associated with bisphosphonate therapy?**

    A. Constipation
    B. Diarrhoea
    C. Increase in creatine kinase
    D. Increase in alanine aminotransferase
    E. Increased risk of eczema

54. **A 57-year-old woman with a BMI of 29 attends clinic for a review of hypertension. Her medication includes ramipril 10 mg od and amlodipine 5 mg od. Her blood pressure remained elevated at 155/90 mmHg and she was started on bendroflumethiazide 2.5 mg od. Which of the following should you warn her is a recognized adverse effect of thiazide therapy?**

    A. Hypocalcaemia
    B. Hypomagnesaemia
    C. Hypouricaemia
    D. Hyperkalaemia
    E. Hyperglycaemia

55. **A 67-year-old woman with a history of hypertension treated with ramipril complained of a chronic dry cough. Her medication was changed to valsartan which resolved her symptoms. Which of the following is most likely to be reduced following this change in medication?**

    A. Angiotensin 1
    B. Angiotensin 2
    C. Bradykinin
    D. Endothelin
    E. Renin

56. **A 64-year-old man has end-stage COPD, his FEV1/FVC is <50% predicted. He has recently stopped smoking. On examination his BP is 155/92, his pulse is 70, atrial fibrillation. There are coarse crackles consistent with COPD on auscultation of the chest. Which of the following medications is most likely to reduce his exacerbation frequency?**

    A. Salbutamol PRN
    B. Atrovent PRN
    C. Oral theophylline
    D. Low-dose inhaled corticosteroids
    E. High-dose inhaled corticosteroids and long-acting beta-2 agonist therapy

57. **Where in the kidney is acetazolamide thought to act?**

    A. Ascending loop of Henlé
    B. Descending loop of Henlé
    C. Proximal convoluted tubule
    D. Proximal portion of distal convoluted tubule
    E. Distal portion of distal convoluted tubule

58. **A 73-year-old woman is discharged from hospital after a left total hip replacement taking rivaroxaban for venous thromboembolism prophylaxis. Which clotting factor is inhibited by rivaroxaban?**

    A. IIa
    B. IX
    C. Xa
    D. XI
    E. XII

59. **A 53-year-old man is reviewed in clinic six weeks after an inferior myocardial infarction. During his admission his total cholesterol was found to be elevated at 6.7 mmol/l and he was started on atorvastatin 20 mg nocte. Unfortunately he suffered multiple muscle aches and his creatine kinase rose to 421 U/l. The statin was discontinued and he was started on ezetimibe. What is the best description of the mode of action of ezetimibe?**

    A. HMG co-A reductase inhibitor
    B. Lipoprotein lipase activator
    C. Lipoprotein lipase inhibitor
    D. NPC1L1 inhibitor
    E. PPAR-gamma agonist

60. **A 41-year-old man comes to the clinic for review of his asthma. He is currently managed with fluticasone 100 mcg BD but still has problems with a cough at night and when he tries to exercise. On examination in the clinic there is only scattered wheeze, but his peak flow is reduced at 410 (530 predicted). You decide to add salmeterol to his regime. Which of the following correctly describes the mode of action of salmeterol?**

    A. Short-acting anti-cholinergic
    B. Potent beta-2 agonist
    C. Long-acting anti-cholinergic
    D. Beta-2 partial agonist
    E. Beta-1 antagonist

61. **A 45-year-old man who has undergone a renal transplant presents to the clinic with symptoms of thirst, polyuria, and gradual weight gain. A random blood sugar reveals a glucose of 9.2 mmol/l and you diagnose him with diabetes mellitus. Which of the following immunosuppressive agents is most likely to have been responsible?**

    A. Ciclosporin
    B. Prednisolone
    C. Azathioprine
    D. Tacrolimus
    E. Sirolimus

62. **A 65-year-old man is reviewed in clinic because of resistant hypertension. His past medical history includes type 2 diabetes and microalbuminuria. He has been intolerant of multiple anti-hypertensive medications and his blood pressure in clinic remains 164/92 mmHg. You are considering starting aliskiren. What is the best description of its mode of action?**

   A. Aldosterone receptor antagonist
   B. Angiotensin 2 converting enzyme antagonist
   C. Renin receptor antagonist
   D. Renin antagonist
   E. Renin activator

63. **You are examining a member of a family that suffers from congenital hypoparathyroidism. You suspect they may carry a mutation of the parathyroid hormone receptor. Which of the following correctly describes the parathyroid hormone receptor?**

   A. G-protein-coupled receptor
   B. Steroid hormone receptor
   C. PPAR-gamma receptor
   D. PPAR-alpha receptor
   E. Voltage-gated ion channel

64. **You are reviewing the results of a new agent for the treatment of epilepsy, but you are concerned that in the one-year pivotal phase 3 study, 4% of patients suffered from a significant rise in blood pressure for the new treatment, versus 2% on the leading existing therapy. Which of the following is the number needed to harm for the new therapy with respect to hypertension?**

   A. 2
   B. 4
   C. 25
   D. 50
   E. 100

65. **One of your patients who is taking part in a diabetes trial comes to the emergency room having suffered a myocardial infarction. He is 56 years old, is treated with metformin and sulphonylurea, and his average HbA1c over the past year has been 8.5%. You are debating how the event should be reported. How should this event be classified?**
    A. Adverse event reported within seven days to the study sponsor
    B. Expected event, no need to report to the sponsor
    C. Serious adverse event, should be reported immediately to the sponsor
    D. Trial endpoint, no need to be reported
    E. Serious adverse event, should be reported within seven days to the sponsor

66. **A 45-year-old car mechanic is admitted having taken an overdose of ethylene glycol and is in an intoxicated state when you review him in the emergency department. You elect to treat him with an infusion of fomepizole. Which of the following is the mode of action of fomepizole?**
    A. Competitive agonist of alcohol dehydrogenase
    B. Non-competitive antagonist of alcohol dehydrogenase
    C. Competitive antagonist of alcohol dehydrogenase
    D. Uncompetitive antagonist of alcohol dehydrogenase
    E. Competitive antagonist of alcohol hydrogenase

67. **A man with COPD who is taking long-term theophylline and combination LABA and steroid inhaler presents to the emergency department with a respiratory tract infection. He is pyrexial 38.2°C. and has a cough productive of purulent sputum. Which of the following antibiotics is likely to be least appropriate for him?**
    A. Ciprofloxacin
    B. Co-amoxiclav
    C. Clarithromycin
    D. Erythromycin
    E. Doxycycline

68. **When thinking about drug metabolism in the liver, which of the following enzyme processes is classified as a phase 1 reaction?**
    A. Glutathione conjugation
    B. Oxidation
    C. Sulphonation
    D. Acetylation
    E. Glucuronidation

69. **A 34-year-old woman was admitted for investigation of dyspnoea. She was found to have pulmonary hypertension. Which of the following findings would be an indication for bosentan therapy?**
    A. PAH secondary to scleroderma with significant interstitial lung disease
    B. Functional class 2 PAH without significant interstitial lung disease
    C. Functional class 3 PAH without significant interstitial lung disease
    D. Functional class 3 PAH where a prostaglandin receptor agonist has failed to control symptoms
    E. Functional class 3 PAH where a phosphodiesterase-5 inhibitor has failed to control symptoms

70. **A 19-year-old woman presents to the emergency department with trismus and torticolis; she looks in absolute agony. Apparently, she has been prescribed an anti-emetic by her GP for persistent vomiting after an episode of food poisoning. Which of the following anti-emetics is the most likely cause?**
    A. Ondansetron
    B. Metaclopramide
    C. Domperidone
    D. Cyclizine
    E. Promethazine

71. **A 51-year-old man was reviewed in the cardiovascular risk clinic. It was decided to add fenofibrate to his treatment regimen. What is the best description of its mode of action?**
    A. Lipoprotein lipase activator
    B. HMG CoA reductase inhibitor
    C. PPAR-delta activator
    D. PPAR-gamma activator
    E. NPC1L1 inhibitor

72. A 47-year-old man presents to the dermatology outpatient clinic complaining of a rash. On examination he has well-demarcated erythematous plaques with associated silver scaling affecting the flexor surfaces of both elbows and knees. A diagnosis of psoriasis is made. His regular medications are listed below. Which one of these medications can cause worsening of psoriasis?

A. Olanzapine
B. Atenolol
C. Ciclosporin
D. Paracetamol
E. Amiodarone

73. A 41-year-old man who has undergone a renal transplant comes to see his GP with a respiratory tract infection and requests antibiotics. His current medication for immunosuppression includes ciclosporin. Which of the following antibiotics is most likely to cause a significant change in his ciclosporin levels?

A. Amoxicillin
B. Clarithromycin
C. Azithromycin
D. Ciprofloxacin
E. Trimethoprim

74. A 72-year-old man was admitted to hospital with increasing exertional breathlessness. His past medical history included an anterior myocardial infarction and heart failure with a left ventricular ejection fraction of 10–15%. During his admission his medication was optimized which improved his breathlessness but he complained that he seems to have 'developed breasts' in recent months. Which of his medications is most likely to be responsible for the development of gynaecomastia?

A. Aspirin
B. Bisoprolol
C. Bumetanide
D. Ramipril
E. Simvastatin

75. You are responsible for drawing up protocols for the management of venous thromboembolus prophylaxis in your hospital. You are aware that rivaroxaban has recently become available. Which of the following correctly describes the mode of action of rivaroxaban?

A. Vitamin K antagonist
B. Factor IX inhibitor
C. Factor Xa inhibitor
D. Factor VIII activator
E. Factor XI inhibitor

76. You decide to start a 54-year-old man who has metastatic colonic carcinoma on a regime that incorporates capecitabine. Which of the following correctly describes the mode of action of capecitabine?

A. It is converted to a pyrimidine analogue
B. It is a pyrimidine analogue
C. It is an alkylating agent
D. It is a nitrogen mustard
E. It is a calcineurin inhibitor

77. You are examining a submission for reimbursement written about a new oral blood glucose lowering agent that has been submitted to the Scottish Medicines consortium. Which of the following types of study is likely to provide the most valuable evidence with respect to determining whether the drug should be reimbursed?

A. Pre-clinical study
B. Phase 1 study
C. Phase 2 study
D. Phase 3 study
E. Phase 4 study

78. You are planning to prescribe a partial opiate agonist for the treatment of opiate withdrawal in one of your patients. Which of the following is a partial opiate agonist?

A. Buprenorphine
B. Codeine
C. Diamorphine
D. Naloxone
E. Flumazenil

79. Bioavailability is a measure of the fraction of an orally administered agent that reaches the plasma. It is related to how polar the administered agent is, and its molecular size. Which of the following agents is known to have the poorest bioavailability?

    A. Risedronate
    B. Simvastatin
    C. Digoxin
    D. Penicillin V
    E. Paracetamol

80. A 48-year-old man is undergoing treatment for tuberculosis with triple combination therapy which includes isoniazid. Unfortunately, he has begun to develop signs of hepatitis and sideroblastic anaemia, and you wonder if he may be predisposed to isoniazid side effects. Which of the following is most likely to be associated with isoniazid toxicity?

    A. Fast acetylation
    B. Slow acetylation
    C. CYP2D6 slow metabolism
    D. CYP2D6 fast metabolism
    E. CYP2C9 polymorphism

81. A 72-year-old man who is taking warfarin for chronic atrial fibrillation presents to the emergency department with easy bruising and bleeding from his gums. Other medication of note includes gliclazide and metformin for type 2 diabetes, and ramipril and indapamide for hypertension. On examination his BP is 122/82, his pulse is 73, atrial fibrillation. He has extensive bruising to his forearms. He has an INR of 7.1. On further questioning he tells you that he has been following a juicing diet that he read about on the Internet. Which of the following fruit juices is likely to have caused his raised INR?

    A. Apple juice
    B. Grapefruit juice
    C. Orange juice
    D. Cranberry juice
    E. Tomato juice

82. **A 51-year-old man is started on metoprolol 50 mg BD for prophylaxis against episodes of paroxysmal atrial fibrillation. Unfortunately he returns to the emergency room only the following day, having taken two doses of the medication, because he has measured his pulse rate at 38 and he feels lightheaded and dizzy. His blood pressure is only 105/60. Which of the following CYP450 enzymes is he likely to be carrying a polymorphism for?**

A. CYP3A4
B. CYP2C8
C. CYP2D6
D. CYP1A2
E. CYP2C9

83. **A 42-year-old man who has undergone a renal transplant some four years previously comes to the emergency room complaining of a sore throat and a fever. Full blood count reveals a marked neutropaenia. Apparently he takes azathioprine as part of his immunosuppressive regime, and has recently visited the emergency GP service complaining of acute gout. Which of the following medications is most likely to have precipitated his acute neutropaenia?**

A. Colchicine
B. Ibuprofen
C. Diclofenac
D. Allopurinol
E. Prednisolone

84. **A 19-year-old student presents with a four-day history of sore throat, headache, fever, and myalgia. He is commenced on oral amoxicillin by his general practitioner. One hour later he presents to the emergency department with a widespread maculopapular rash. His breathing is laboured with an audible wheeze. Blood pressure is 90/40 mmHg, heart rate 105 bpm, RR 32/min and SpO$_2$ 96% on air. What should the next management step be?**

A. Change amoxicillin to penicillin V
B. Change amoxicillin to aciclovir
C. Give high flow oxygen and 0.5 ml 1:1000 adrenaline IM
D. Give high flow oxygen and 0.5 ml of 1:10,000 adrenaline IV
E. Give high flow oxygen and nebulized salbutamol

85. **A 70-year-old white man with ANCA-associated vasculitis previously treated with multiple courses of cyclophosphamide, currently in drug-free remission, has persistent microscopic haematuria on three consecutive occasions a month apart. There is no pain or proteinuria, and a renal ultrasound is normal. His blood tests show normal inflammatory markers, and the urea, electrolytes, and creatinine have been stable for the last two years. What is the next step in his management?**
   A. Biopsy of kidneys
   B. CT renal angiogram
   C. Cystoscopy
   D. Intravenous urogram
   E. Urine culture for TB

86. **A 56-year-old woman is reviewed for hypertension. Her medication includes bendroflumethiazide 2.5 mg od. On examination her blood pressure is 136/76 mmHg. Investigations: Biochemistry: sodium 138 mmol/l , potassium 3.1 mmol/l, creatinine 81 micromol/l. What is the most likely cause of her hypokalaemia?**
   A. Increased sodium in the proximal segment of the distal tubule
   B. Increased sodium in the distal segment of the distal tubule
   C. Increased potassium in the proximal segment of the distal tubule
   D. Increased potassium in the distal segment of the distal tubule
   E. Increased sodium in the collecting duct

87. **A 69-year-old man was anti-coagulated with warfarin following a pulmonary embolus. His INR had previously been very stable; however, on this occasion it was 4.3. He reported taking co-enzyme Q10, an 'antibiotic' for 'a stomach infection', and stated that he had been out a couple of days previously to celebrate his birthday. Which of the following would be safest to continue in the light of his INR increase?**
   A. Ciprofloxacin
   B. Co-enzyme Q10 supplements
   C. Fluconazole
   D. Increased alcohol consumption
   E. Metronidazole

88. **A 26-year-old woman presents with syncope. She reports a three-month history of increasing shortness of breath since the birth of her first child.I nvestigations: Echocardiography: normal left and right ventricular function, pulmonary hypertension with a PA pressure calculated at 70 mmHg. It is elected to start her on bosentan. What is the best description of its mode of action?**
    A. Endothelin A receptor antagonist
    B. Endothelin receptor antagonist
    C. Endothelin A and B receptor antagonist
    D. Endothelin A receptor agonist
    E. Endothelin B receptor agonist

89. **A 68-year-old man is admitted following a suspected significant overdose of propranolol which he has been prescribed for agitation. He reports lethargy and light-headedness. On examination he is alert and orientated with a regular pulse of 44 bpm and a blood pressure of 140/88 mmHg. What is the most appropriate initial management?**
    A. Adenosine
    B. Glucagon
    C. Isoprenaline
    D. Magnesium
    E. Transvenous temporary pacing

90. **A 63-year-old man was reviewed in the outpatient clinic. He had permanent atrial fibrillation and was taking digoxin 125 mcg od which he tolerated well. Unfortunately, he had been intolerant of multiple other medications to control his ventricular rate which remained >110 bpm. You have decided to add a further medication to his regimen but want to avoid increasing his plasma digoxin concentration. Which drug is least likely to increase his plasma concentration of digoxin?**
    A. Amiodarone
    B. Atenolol
    C. Propafenone
    D. Quinidine
    E. Verapamil

91. **A 69-year-old woman with long-standing COPD comes to the emergency department with severe nausea and vomiting. She takes a seretide inhaler, tiotropium, and theophylline tablets, and tells you she was prescribed an antibiotic by the on-call GP two nights earlier. On examination her BP is 145/72, her pulse is 95. Her respiratory rate is 20 with bilateral scattered wheeze. Which of the following antibiotics is most likely to have contributed to her presentation?**

A. Amoxicillin
B. Azithromycin
C. Ciprofloxacin
D. Trimethoprim
E. Doxycycline

92. **A 28-year-old man is admitted with a tachycardia and severe agitation. He reports going to a night club and taking three lines of cocaine. On examination he has a regular pulse of 140 bpm and a blood pressure of 155/90 mmHg. His chest was clear to auscultation. Investigations: ECG: narrow complex tachycardia at 140 bpm. What is the best treatment for his arrhythmia?**

A. Amiodarone
B. Bisoprolol
C. Digoxin
D. Flecainide
E. Verapamil

93. **A 27-year-old woman is admitted to the emergency department with acute severe asthma. Her peak flow on admission to the unit is 150 (normal 510). She usually takes BD seretide 125/25 and monteleukast and has had two previous admissions to the ITU. You give her continuous salbutamol nebulizers, an ipratropium nebulizer, and IV hydrocortisone, but 30 mins later her peak flow has only improved to 210. Which of the following is the next most appropriate intervention?**

A. Intravenous aminophylline
B. Intravenous salbutamol
C. Intravenous magnesium sulphate
D. NIPPV
E. Intravenous chlorpheniramine

94. **A 62-year-old man is admitted with symptoms of phenytoin toxicity, including diplopia, nystagmus, and ataxia. He takes the phenytoin for tonic clonic seizures and has done for many years. He has suffered a severe diarrhoeal illness over the past few days. Routine bloods are taken: haemoglobin 13.1 g/dl (13.5–17.7), white cells 10.1 x 10⁹/l (4–11), platelets 207 x 10⁹/l (150–400), sodium 139 mmol/l (135–146), potassium 5.4 mmol/l (3.5–5), creatinine 237 micromol/l (79–118), phenytoin 17 mg/l (10–20). Why does he have symptoms of phenytoin toxicity?**

A. Decreased phenytoin protein binding
B. Increased phenytoin protein binding
C. Decreased phenytoin excretion
D. Decreased serum albumin
E. Increased serum pH

95. **A 46-year-old woman who has a history of anxiety and depression is brought to the emergency department having been found unconscious by her neighbour with an empty bottle of diazepam 5 mg tablets. On examination you cannot wake her, her BP is 100/60 and her pulse is 78. Her respiratory rate is 8 and her pupils are dilated. How would you manage her?**

A. Intravenous flumazenil
B. Intravenous naloxone
C. Intubation and ventilation
D. Intravenous glucagon
E. Subcutaneous adrenalin

96. **A 42-year-old man with anxiety has been taking fluoxetine for many years. He is now in a stable job and feels he would like to stop the medication. He has heard about SSRI withdrawal on the internet. Which of the following is true of SSRI withdrawal?**

A. Symptoms invariably only last for a few days
B. Feelings of depersonalization are seen
C. Constipation is common
D. Stopping the medication abruptly is unlikely to cause a problem in the majority of patients
E. He is likely to suffer from hypersomnia

97. A 62-year-old woman is admitted unconscious by ambulance after being found by her son. She has long-term problems with anxiety and takes regular diazepam from her GP. Her son returned home from an evening out to find an empty bottle of wine and two empty bottles of diazepam 5 mg tablets. On examination her BP is 85/50, her pulse 82, and her pupils are dilated. She is unconscious and there is vomit around the corner of her mouth. Which of the following is the most appropriate treatment for her?

A. Fomepizole
B. Flumazenil
C. Naloxone
D. Intubation and ventilation
E. Haemofiltration

98. A 63-year-old patient with active rheumatoid arthritis comes to the clinic for review. You wish to start her on a non-steroidal anti-inflammatory agent, but she has a past history of indigestion. When reviewing the relative risk of GI adverse events associated with their use, which of the following non-steroidals has the highest risk?

A. Diclofenac IR
B. Diclofenac SR
C. Naproxen
D. Ibuprofen
E. Ketoprofen

99. A 71-year-old is admitted to the ITU with enterobacter septicaemia. You elect to treat her with imipenem as part of her antibiotic regime. Which of the following is true of imipenem?

A. It does not normally penetrate inflamed meninges
B. It has high oral bioavailability
C. Dose modification is not required in renal failure
D. It binds to penicillin binding protein
E. There is no cross reactivity with penicillin

100. **A 22-year-old student presents to the university health service complaining of a watery grey offensive smelling vaginal discharge that she says has a fishy odour. She has had one sexual partner over the past six months and tells you that they have used condoms. On examination the vulval skin looks normal, but you confirm a thin, grey white discharge which emits a strong fishy smell on mixing with potassium hydroxide. Which of the following is most appropriate treatment for her?**

A. Clotrimazole cream
B. Ciprofloxacin
C. Metronidazole
D. Co-amoxiclav
E. Azithromycin

101. **A 56-year-old man suffers persistent nausea after receiving IV diamorphine for chest pain related to an anterior myocardial infarction. You elect to prescribe cyclizine for his nausea. Which of the following correctly describes the mode of action of cyclizine?**

A. H2 receptor antagonism
B. H1 receptor antagonism
C. D1 receptor antagonism
D. D2 receptor antagonism
E. 5-HT2 receptor antagonism

102. **Which of the following drugs used to treat infection with *Mycobacterium tuberculosis* is least likely to be associated with hepatotoxicity?**

A. Ethambutol
B. Isoniazid
C. Pyrazinamide
D. Rifampicin
E. All of the above are recognized causes of hepatotoxicity

103. **A 61-year-old woman with a history of rheumatoid arthritis, a previous stroke, and a duodenal ulcer comes to the clinic for review. Medication of note includes ramipril, atorvastatin, and low-dose aspirin. She takes paracetamol intermittently for pain from her rheumatoid arthritis and takes methotrexate once weekly. She is requesting diclofenac to relieve her pain. Which of the following best reflects the NICE advice with respect to use of NSAIDs in this case?**

A. The lowest dose of NSAID to control symptoms should be used

B. Ibuprofen should be the initial NSAID used

C. Omeprazole should always be started with the NSAID

D. Misoprostol should always be started with the NSAID

E. Ranitidine should always be started with the NSAID

104. **Regarding nucleoside reverse transcriptase inhibitors for the treatment of HIV (such as zidovudine), which of the following is not a recognized side effect?**

A. Lactic acidosis

B. Lipodystrophy

C. Macrocytosis

D. Myopathy

E. QT prolongation

105. **You review a patient with metastatic carcinoma of the breast, and determine that she is suitable for lapatinib therapy. Which of the following correctly describes a feature of lapatanib?**

A. Inhibitor of ErbB1 and ErbB2 receptors

B. Inhibitor of HER-2 receptors

C. Inhibitor of oestrogen receptors

D. Inhibitor of progesterone receptors

E. Inhibitor of platelet-derived growth factor receptors

106. **A young woman with rheumatoid arthritis is started on methotrexate. She says she might consider starting a family in a couple of years or so. What advice would you give her?**

A. You have no concerns about her becoming pregnant whilst on methotrexate

B. She should stop methotrexate once she has a positive pregnancy test

C. She should stop methotrexate at least three months prior to trying for a baby

D. She should never take methotrexate if she wants a family in the future

E. Not enough is known about effects in pregnancy to make a recommendation

107. A 34-year-old pregnant woman with a BMI of 29 presents to the GP midwife for a 24-week check and is found to have glycosuria. This is her second pregnancy. Her first pregnancy was unremarkable apart from the fact that the child was nearly 11 lb in weight. On examination, BP is 115/75, pulse is 70, the remainder of the examination is unremarkable. Investigations: haemoglobin 11.6 g/dl (11.5–16.5), white cell count 5.1 x $10^9/l$ (4–11), platelets 198 x $10^9/l$ (150–400), serum sodium 142 mmol/l (135–146), serum potassium 4.2 mmol/l (3.5–5), creatinine 98 micromol/l (79–118), fasting plasma glucose 7.5 mmol/l post diet and exercise. Which of the following is the most appropriate way to manage her?

A. Glibenclamide
B. Basal insulin
C. Basal bolus insulin
D. Pioglitazone
E. Metformin

108. A 42-year-old man is involved in a road traffic accident and suffers an open fracture of his tibia and fibula. He is initially stabilized with fluid resuscitation and is given a tetanus booster whilst awaiting orthopaedic surgery. A few minutes later the nurses notice that his BP has dropped by 20 mmHg, his pulse has increased to 95, and he has erythema around the tetanus booster site. This responded to more fluids, SC adrenalin and IV corticosteroids. Patch testing in the outpatients department a few weeks later shows hypersensitivity to tetanus toxoid. Which of the following types of hypersensitivity reaction is this?

A. Type 1
B. Type 2
C. Type 3
D. Type 4
E. Type 5

109. A 52-year-old man complains of an itchy, scaly rash affecting his scalp and the extensor surfaces of both arms. He has recently begun a number of cardiovascular medications after an admission with an NSTEMI. On examination he has a typical psoriatic rash. Which of the following medications is most likely to have been responsible?

A. Isosorbide dinitrate
B. Atorvastatin
C. Bisoprolol
D. Indapamide
E. Clopidogrel

110. **You are examining the potential for a new oral antibiotic to be used for the treatment of otitis media. One determinant of effectiveness is the time taken for the new drug to reach its maximum plasma concentration. Which of the following is likely to impact most on the T-max of this new agent?**
    A. Absorption
    B. Distribution
    C. Metabolism
    D. Excretion
    E. Dose administered

111. **A 78-year-old man is admitted to the ward with marked lethargy, confusion, and acute renal failure. Following a poor-quality ultrasound, the urology team book an urgent CT scan with contrast which is also not diagnostic. Following the scan, the patient's renal function deteriorates further. The team are alerted to the fact that metformin (2000 mg daily) and various other nephrotoxic agents have remained on the patient's prescription. Which of the following regarding the pharmacology of metformin is correct?**
    A. The drug undergoes liver metabolism
    B. In the absence of renal impairment, the drug has a plasma half-life of 12–18 hours
    C. The drug has a bioavailability of 80%
    D. The drug is transported bound to plasma proteins
    E. The drug has no known metabolites

112. **You are reviewing the results of a phase 1 study of a new anti-hypertensive drug. Maximal plasma concentration of 20 nmol/l is reached 2 hours after administration. At four hours after administration this has fallen to 15 nmol/l. What is the half-life of this new agent?**
    A. Two hours
    B. Four hours
    C. Six hours
    D. Eight hours
    E. Ten hours

113. **A 70-year-old woman has a four-month history of a dry pruritic rash affecting the upper back and shins. Which is the most appropriate initial management of this patient?**

A. Avoid contact irritants

B. Use emollients

C. Skin biopsy

D. Use topical corticosteroids

E. A history is needed to ascertain the contact allergen

114. **A 52-year-old man is started on ramipril for the treatment of hypertension by his GP. He is concerned about possible side effects of therapy. Which of the following is commonly reported in conjunction with ramipril treatment?**

A. Angioedema

B. Dry cough

C. Impotence

D. Rash

E. Gout

115. **You are attempting to develop a new drug to prevent worsening of diabetic nephropathy. You want it to have a low level of first-pass metabolism as it has a direct action in animal models on the glomerular basement membrane. When considering drugs and first-pass metabolism, which agent has the lowest first-pass metabolism?**

A. Propranolol

B. Chlorpromazine

C. Levodopa

D. Isosorbide dinitrate

E. Digoxin

116. **A 71-year-old man with a history of COPD comes to the emergency room with nausea and vomiting. He is taking high-dose seretide and theophylline tablets for control of his chest disease. Most recently he consulted an emergency GP who prescribed an antibiotic, although he is unaware of the name of this. On examination his BP is 122/72, he is tachycardic with a pulse of 105. Which of the following antibiotics is most likely to be related to his symptoms?**

    A. Amoxicillin
    B. Ciprofloxacin
    C. Azithromycin
    D. Co-amoxiclav
    E. Penicillin V

117. **A 69-year-old woman is taking simvastatin, ramipril, and indapamide after a previous myocardial infarction. She is also being treated for tuberculosis. She presents to her GP complaining of muscle ache, tiredness, and lethargy. On examination she has calf tenderness to deep palpation. You find her to have a raised CK of 720 on laboratory testing. Which of the following is most likely to be the cause of her presentation?**

    A. Cranberry juice
    B. Grapefruit juice
    C. Rifampicin
    D. Isoniazid
    E. Indapamide

118. **A patient on your ward with a metallic mitral valve is found to have an INR of 1.4. It was previously stable at 3–4. Which of his recently started medications is most likely to have caused this?**

    A. Ciprofloxacin
    B. Omeprazole
    C. Rifampicin
    D. Erythromycin
    E. Allopurinol

119. A 47-year-old man with bipolar disorder, who is maintained on long-term lithium therapy, presents to casualty feeling generally unwell. He gives a 4-day history of nausea, vomiting, and loose stools. On examination he has a coarse tremor, is globally weak, and struggles with visual acuity due to blurring of his vision. Lithium toxicity is suspected and subsequently confirmed with blood testing. On further questioning it appears he was started on a new medication for hypertension approximately one week prior to his presentation. Which one of the following medications is the most likely culprit in this case of lithium toxicity?

A. Doxazosin
B. Methyldopa
C. Bendroflumethiazide
D. Atenolol
E. Amlodipine

120. A 34-year-old woman with a history of diabetes presents with worsening jaundice. She is being treated with a second course of oral antibiotics for a urinary tract infection. Her liver function tests show her bilirubin is 64 µmol/l, ALT is 54 IU/l, AST is 67 IU/l, and ALP 208 IU/l. Which of the following medications is least likely to be the cause of her abnormal liver biochemistry?

A. Co-amoxiclav
B. Nitrofurantoin
C. Microgynon (combined oral contraceptive pill)
D. Atorvastatin
E. Gliclazide

121. An 89-year-old man was admitted with a 24-hour history of confusion and drowsiness. He had a history of alcohol excess, type 2 diabetes mellitus, arthritis, hypertension, and carcinoma of the colon with right hemi-colectomy and colostomy. He was taking bendroflumethiazide 2.5 mg daily, amlodipine 5 mg daily, and codeine 15 mg QDS prn. Serum sodium was 114 mmol/l and so bendroflumethiazide was stopped and serum sodium corrected over the next five days. He was also started on chlordiazepoxide for alcohol detoxification and enoxaparin for thromboprophylaxis. Blood results one week and three weeks after admission were as shown in Table 4.1. Which drug was most likely to be responsible for the hyperkalaemia.

A. Amlodipine
B. Bendroflumethiazide
C. Chlordiazepoxide
D. Codeine
E. Enoxaparin

Table 4.1 Blood results

	One week	Three weeks
Reference Hb (13–18 g/dl)	14.6 g/dl	13.8 g/dl
WBC (4–11 × 10⁹/l)	7.6 × 10⁹/l	6.8 × 10⁹/l
Platelets (150–400 × 10⁹/l)	177 × 10⁹/l	201 × 10⁹/l
Na (137–144 mmol/l)	136 mmol/l	142 mmol/l
K (3.5–4.9 mmol/l)	5.1 mmol/l	5.8 mmol/l
Urea (2.5–7.0 mmol/l)	6.4 mmol/l	6.6 mmol/l
Creatinine (60–110 micromol/l)	99 micromol/l	106 micromol/l

122. **All of the following are potential side effects of gentamicin except:**
    A. Hepatic impairment
    B. Hypomagnesaemia
    C. Ototoxicity
    D. Renal impairment
    E. Stomatitis

123. **You are looking at the study programme for a new drug to treat type 2 diabetes mellitus. The programme is designed to test safety in healthy volunteers, dose ranging in subjects with diabetes, and then clinical efficacy, and finally health outcome measures. Where is dose ranging normally tested in a clinical trial programme?**
    A. Phase 1
    B. Phase 2
    C. Phase 3
    D. Phase 4
    E. Real-life database study

124. **A new antibiotic is launched for the treatment of lower respiratory tract infection. There is increasing concern, however, as a number of yellow cards have been received with respect to supraventricular tachycardias associated with its use. Which of the following is the body required to make decisions with respect to the safety of this drug in the UK?**
    A. NICE
    B. Scottish Medicines Consortium
    C. Department of Health
    D. MHRA
    E. Hospital prescribing committees

125. **A 55-year-old man is found to be in atrial fibrillation during a routine medical insurance consultation. He does not describe a history of syncope, palpitations, or shortness of breath. His past medical history is otherwise unremarkable. After a lengthy discussion, he has decided not to undergo cardioversion. If the patient remains in rate-controlled atrial fibrillation, which is the best treatment option for him?**
    A. Warfarin, target INR 2–3
    B. No anticoagulation
    C. Warfarin target INR 2–3 for 6 months then aspirin
    D. Digoxin
    E. Aspirin

126. **You are interested in doing a trial with a drug that is commonly used for blood pressure, because you believe that it may have activity against breast cancer. You are reviewing what paperwork needs to be submitted to the MHRA (Medicines Regulatory Agency) before beginning the study. Which of the following is an essential part of the documentation?**
    A. CTA (clinical trial application)
    B. IND (investigational new drug application)
    C. Yellow card
    D. BLA (biological licence application)
    E. NICE submission

127. **What would be considered the first-line antiepileptic medication for absence seizures?**
    A. Phenytoin
    B. Carbamazepine
    C. Topiramate
    D. Levetiracetam
    E. Sodium valproate

128. **Which of the following drug combinations is not recognized to cause a significant interaction?**
    A. Calcium + vitamin D supplements and levothyroxine
    B. Methotrexate and trimethoprim
    C. Clarithromycin and simvastatin
    D. Clopidogrel and omeprazole
    E. Doxazosin and carbamazepine

129. A 56-year-old man with a history of symptomatic gout comes to the clinic for review of his blood pressure control. He has recently been started on losartan 100mg daily, and notices that his gout has improved. There has been a corresponding 30% reduction in his serum urate. How does losartan therapy lead to a fall in serum urate?

A. Inhibition of URAT-1
B. Inhibition of intracellular microtubules
C. Inhibition of xanthine oxidase
D. Uricase activator
E. Uricase inhibitor

130. A 17-year-old woman presents to the emergency room severely agitated. She is staring into space and is complaining of neck stiffness and jaw spasm. She had an episode of food poisoning after a take-away curry, and took an anti-emetic given to her by a friend who has a history of migraine. Apparently these symptoms came on very soon after taking the tablet. On examination she has evidence of torticollis, a fixed stare and is severely agitated. Which of the following antiemetics is she most likely to have taken?

A. Cyclizine
B. Domperidone
C. Metaclopramide
D. Ondansetron
E. Promethazine

131. A 28-year-old man is brought to the emergency department by ambulance, having ingested 10 g of sodium valproate some three hours earlier after a row with his girlfriend. He is very drowsy with a GCS of 13 on admission. His BP is 100/60 with a pulse of 90. Routine U&E and FBC are normal, as is CXR. Which of the following is the most appropriate way to manage him?

A. Gastric lavage
B. Oral activated charcoal
C. Ipecac
D. Haemodialysis
E. Supportive therapy only

132. **You are performing a PEG insertion on a 71-year-old woman with a left hemiplegia and unsafe swallow after an ischaemic stroke. She is given midazolam for sedation and initially tolerates the procedure well, maintaining saturations of 93%. The nurse asks you to stop as her respiratory rate has fallen to 8, and her O2 saturation to 87%. The nurse begins to bag her. Which of the following is the most appropriate next intervention?**

    A. Flumazenil
    B. Naloxone
    C. Glucagon
    D. Continue bag and mask until the midazolam wears off
    E. Doxapram

133. **You are examining the properties of a new agent for the treatment of schizophrenia. It is highly lipid soluble. Which of the following is likely to be true with respect to its properties?**

    A. It is likely to be excreted unchanged by the kidney
    B. It is likely to have a large volume of distribution
    C. It is likely to be very soluble in plasma
    D. It is likely to be very soluble in infusion solutions
    E. It is likely to have a very long plasma half life

134. **A 29-year-old woman with manic depressive psychosis is admitted by ambulance to the emergency department after taking a substantial overdose of lithium tablets. Her GCS is 10 on admission, with a BP of 100/60 and a pulse of 105. Her sodium measured on the blood gas analyser is 134 mmol/L, and an urgent lithium level is reported by the lab to be 4.3 mmol/L. Which of the following represents the optimal management in this case?**

    A. Whole bowel irrigation
    B. Activated charcoal
    C. Haemodialysis
    D. Forced alkaline diuresis
    E. Induced vomiting

135. **A 70-year-old gardener is brought to the emergency department by his daughter. He admitted to her that he drank a quantity of paraquat weedkiller some four hours earlier. You estimate that he has consumed some 12 g of paraquat. What is the likelihood that the ingested dose is fatal?**

A. 0%

B. 10%

C. 25%

D. 50%

E. 100%

136. **You are developing a new agent for the treatment of blood pressure. When examining its pharmacokinetic properties, which of the following is most likely to preclude its successful development?**

A. Half life of nine hours

B. High molecular weight

C. High degree of polarity

D. 20% renal excretion

E. CYP 2C9 metabolism

137. **A 65-year-old man with a history of type 2 diabetes and hypertension comes to the vascular prevention clinic for review. He is noted to have a history of atrial fibrillation which is rate controlled on 125 mcg of digoxin and has been present for at least a year. He travels frequently to Pakistan to visit relatives and is reluctant to take warfarin because of difficulties in monitoring. Which of the following is the most appropriate option for prevention of stroke/systemic embolism in this case?**

A. Aspirin 75 mg

B. Aspirin 75 mg and clopidogrel 75 mg

C. Aspirin 300 mg

D. Warfarin therapy with alterations to lifestyle to allow monitoring

E. Dabigatran 150 mg BD

138. **A 21-year-old woman comes for review having suffered a second fit, a generalized tonic clonic seizure. A CT scan has been reported as normal. Medication of note includes the oral contraceptive pill. On examination her BP is 110/72, pulse is 72 and regular. Her BMI is 24. She is very body conscious and is concerned about putting weight on with anti-epileptics. Which of the following medications would be most suitable for her?**

    A. Retigabine
    B. Lamotrigine
    C. Valproate
    D. Carbamazepine
    E. Phenytoin

CLINICAL PHARMACOLOGY, THERAPEUTICS, AND TOXICOLOGY

ANSWERS

1. B. Inhibits the co-transport of Na$^+$/K$^+$/2Cl$^-$ in the thick ascending limb of the loop of Henlé

Loop diuretics block the co-transport of Na$^+$/K$^+$/2Cl$^-$ in the thick ascending limb of the loop of Henle. Thiazides inhibit NaCl transport in the distal convoluted tubule. Amiloride blocks sodium channels in the collecting tubules. Mannitol of course promotes osmotic diuresis.

Longmore M et al., *Oxford Handbook of Clinical Medicine*, Eighth Edition, Oxford University Press, 2010, Chapter 7, Renal medicine, Diuretics and their mechanism of action.

2. A. Carbimazole

This woman has type 1 amiodarone-induced thyroiditis (AIT), which occurs in patients who in all likelihood have a predisposition for autoimmune thyroid disease. Positive thyroid autoantibodies are therefore a feature. Carbimazole is eventually effective but it may take up to two months; potassium perchlorate may be used to gain more rapid control of thyroid disease. Amiodarone should be stopped if possible, but in this case an alternative intervention will be required first.

Richards D et al., *Oxford Handbook of Practical Drug Therapy*, Second Edition, Oxford University Press, 2011, Chapter 2, Cardiovascular system, Antiarrhythmic Drugs: Amiodarone.

3. C. Intubation and ventilation

This patient has had a significant overdose of benzodiazepines and alcohol and is therefore at high risk with respect to not protecting his airway and aspiration. Given that he is a chronic user of temazepam, flumazenil may precipitate seizures and should be avoided. As such the most appropriate option is intubation and ventilation.

Wyatt J et al., *Oxford Handbook of Emergency Medicine*, Fourth Edition, Oxford University Press, 2012, Chapter 4, Toxicology, Benzodiazepine poisoning.

4. A. DNA crosslinking

Alkylating agents exert their biological activity via their ability to covalently bind and crosslink a variety of macromolecules including DNA, RNA, and proteins. They covalently link an alkyl group (R-CH2) to a chemical species in nucleic acids or proteins. This results in impaired DNA replication and transcription, ultimately leading to either cell death or altered cellular function. Alkylating agents includes cyclophosphamide, chlorambucil, busulfan, melphalan, and nitrogen mustard. Vincristine is a vinca alkaloid that is a plant-derived cytotoxic agent whose mechanism of action involves antimicrotubule activity. Methotrexate competitively inhibits dihydrofolate reductase and acts as a folic acid antagonist. Fluorouracil is a pyrimidine analogue resembling pyrimidine molecules and works by inhibiting the synthesis of nucleic acids. Fludarabine is a purine nucleoside analogue (PNA).

Cassidy J et al., *Oxford Handbook of Oncology*, Third Edition, Oxford University Press, 2010, Chapter 6, Principles of chemotherapy, Alkylating agents.

5. A. VEGFR, PDGFR, and c-kit

Pazopanib is an orally administered, potent multi-target tyrosine kinase inhibitor (TKI) of vascular endothelial growth factor receptors (VEGFR)-1, -2, and -3, platelet-derived growth factor (PDGFR-alpha and PDGFR-beta) and stem cell factor receptor (c-KIT). As such it is being investigated for the treatment of a range of solid tumours, but initially it is licensed in the treatment of renal cell carcinoma. Side effects include vomiting, diarrhoea, and mucositis.

McCormack PL, Pazopanib: a review of its use in the management of advanced renal cell carcinoma, *Drugs* 2014 Jul;74(10):1111–1125. doi: 10.1007/s40265-014-0243-3.

6. B. Gastric lavage

Where paraquat has been ingested within one hour of presentation, then gastric lavage is indicated. After this time, activated charcoal is recommended as an option. Urine can be analysed for paraquat levels and this is directly reflective of prognosis. Analgesia may also be considered as the burning sensation caused by paraquat is usually severe. If large enough quantities are ingested, death results from respiratory failure within 7–14 days.

Wyatt J et al., *Oxford Handbook of Emergency Medicine*, Fourth Edition, Oxford University Press, 2012, Chapter 4, Toxicology, Paraquat poisoning.

7. E. Arrange an S1 spinal block

Given that this patient is already on a relatively high dose of morphine, and has significant renal impairment, options for systemic pain relief are very limited. As such, given the pain is limited to the S1 dermatome, a nerve block is likely to be the most effective option. A tunnelled catheter delivering bupivacaine is the usual choice.

Wyatt J et al., *Oxford Handbook of Emergency Medicine*, Fourth Edition, Oxford University Press, 2012, Chapter 7, Analgesia and anaesthesia, General principles of local anaesthesia.

8. D. Prednisolone 40 mg

This clinical picture fits best with sarcoidosis as the most likely cause of hypercalcaemia. As such, high-dose corticosteroids are the most appropriate therapy for lowering the patient's serum calcium. Hypercalcaemia is dependent on reserves of vitamin D to be hydroxylated within granulomata as such patients with sarcoidosis often present after foreign holidays in the sun. Chloroquine and ketoconazole may also reduce vitamin D and may have value as additive therapies. Finally, third-line therapy does involve use of bisphosphonates.

Turner H, Wass J, *Oxford Handbook of Endocrinology and Diabetes*, Second Edition, Oxford University Press, 2009, Part 6: Calcium and bone metabolism, Hypercalcaemia, sarcoidosis.

9. C. Alcohol dehydrogenase inhibitor

Ethylene glycol is first metabolized to glycolaldehyde which then undergoes further oxidation to glycolate, glyoxylate, and oxalate. It is glycolate and oxalate that are primarily responsible for the metabolic acidosis and renal damage that are seen in ethylene glycol poisoning. Fomepizole or 4-methylpyrazole is indicated for use as an antidote in confirmed or suspected methanol or ethylene glycol poisoning. It may be used alone or in combination with haemodialysis. Fomepizole is a competitive inhibitor of alcohol dehydrogenase, the enzyme that catalyses the initial steps in the metabolism of ethylene glycol and methanol to their toxic metabolites. HMG-CoA reductase (or 3-hydroxy-3-methyl-glutaryl-CoA reductase) is the rate-controlling enzyme of the mevalonate pathway, the metabolic pathway that produces cholesterol and other isoprenoids. Statins inhibit HMG-CoA reductase. Allopurinol inhibits xanthine oxidase enzymes and reduces uric acid production. Cyclo-oxygenase (COX) enzyme inhibitors include aspirin and other NSAIDs, and block the formation of important biological mediators called prostanoids, including prostaglandins, prostacyclin, and thromboxane. Digoxin binds to a site on the extracellular aspect of the subunit of the Na/K ATPase pump in the membranes of heart cells, increasing the length of the action potential and reducing heart rate.

Brent J, Fomepizole for ethylene glycol and methanol poisoning, *New England Journal of Medicine* Med 2009;360(21):2216–2223.

10. E. Mycophenolate

Mycophenolate is recognized as causing a Crohn's-like enterocolitis. Patients present with diarrhoea and are found on endoscopy to have Crohn's-like ulceration with skip lesions. Withdrawal of mycophenolate leads to resolution of symptoms over the course of a few weeks.

Dost D et al., Crohn's-like enterocolitis associated with mycophenolic acid treatment, *Gut* 2008;57:1330.

11. C. In the acute setting it is important to test her blood glucose level, electrolytes, and carbamazepine levels

Status epilepticus if defined by either (1) a continuous seizure lasting >30 minutes or (2) intermittent seizures where consciousness is not regained between discrete episodes which last >30 minutes. All patients should have 100% oxygen via non-rebreather mask and a bedside blood glucose should be done. Lorazepam is the first line in drug therapy although diazepam may be used. Second-line treatment of phenytoin is initiated if there is still seizure activity after 10 minutes of having the benzodiazepines. If the patient still has seizure activity after this has been administered, the patient should be transferred to an intensive care setting and intubated. Bloods should be sent to investigate the cause of the prolonged seizure; these should include FBC, U&Es, glucose, calcium, magnesium, LFTs, and a carbamazepine level. If indicated, blood should also be sent for toxicology screen.

Allman K et al., *Emergencies in Anaesthesia*, Second Edition, Oxford University Press, 2006, Chapter 6, Neurosurgery, Status epilepticus.

12. B. Sirolimus

Sirolimus acts via mTOR inhibition and blocks calcium-independent signalling via CD28. This is in contrast to ciclosporin and tacrolimus, which inhibit IL2 production. Cyclosporin A also interferes with B-cell function and antibody production. A range of side effects are associated with sirolimus therapy; these include impaired glucose tolerance and ype 2 diabetes, which has prompted development of alternative regimes of immunosuppression in patients with diabetes mellitus who undergo transplant.

Rapamune prescribing information. http://www.medicines.org.uk/emc/medicine/5747/SPC/Rapamune/#UNDESIRABLE_EFFECTS.

13. A. Ciclosporin toxicity

Ketoconazole is a potent CYP 450 3A4 inhibitor, and as such it promotes accumulation of ciclosporin, leading to toxicity. Macrolide antibiotics, verapamil, diltiazem, amiodarone, and protease inhibitors are also all also known to increase ciclosporin levels and may precipitate toxicity. If these drugs must be prescribed and there are no alternatives, consultation with the transplant physicians is essential so that the ciclosporin can be appropriately down-titrated.

Spickett G, *Oxford Handbook of Clinical Immunology and Allergy*, Second Edition, Oxford University Press, 2006, Chapter 16, Immunotherapy, Immunosuppressive/immunomodulatory drugs: ciclosporin (CyA)/tacrolimus (FK506)/sirolimus (rapamycin).

14. A. Hypoglycaemia

All the answers in the list are potential side effects except hypoglycaemia. Steroids can lead to decreased glucose tolerance with an increased risk of hyperglycaemia and diabetes. It is vital to know about the side effects of steroids, as they are still commonly used for a huge range of conditions. It is important to warn the patient about these effects so that they can make an informed decision about whether to take the medication. It is also important to think about limiting the side effects, for example by using gastric and bone protection when a patient is on prolonged treatment.

BNF, Section 6.3.2, Glucocorticoid therapy. Subsection: Side-effects of corticosteroids. http://www.evidence.nhs.uk/formulary/bnf/current/6-endocrine-system/63-corticosteroids/632-glucocorticoid-therapy/side-effects-of-corticosteroids.

15. A. Thiopurine methyltransferase (TPMT) levels

TPMT is one of the enzymes involved in the metabolism of azathioprine. Individuals can have varying levels of enzyme activity due to genetic differences. If there is a deficiency in this enzyme then individuals are more susceptible to serious complications such as bone marrow failure. COMT is an enzyme that metabolizes catecholamines in the body. Anti-tTG antibodies are often raised in coeliac disease, and so they are tested when this condition is suspected to aid the diagnosis. HLA B27 is a genotype associated with a group of arthropathies including ankylosing spondylitis and enteropathic arthritis. The test for HLA B27 may be carried out to aid the diagnosis of these conditions. Faecal calprotectin testing is a relatively new test to aid in the diagnosis of inflammatory bowel disease.

TPMT testing before azathioprine therapy? *DTB (Drug and Therapeutics Bulletin)* 2009;47:9–12.

16. B. Azithromycin single dose

The optimal treatment of syphilis is is 2.4 MU of IM penicillin, with single-dose azithromycin as the second choice in a penicillin-allergic patient. Doxycycline given as a 14-day course is the third alternative for treatment. Ceftriaxone IM may be used as an alternative to penicillin in pregnant women with allergy. It is also crucial to screen this patient for other sexually transmitted disease.

Eddleston M et al., *Oxford Handbook of Tropical Medicine*, Third Edition, Oxford University Press, 2008, Chapter 16, Sexually transmitted infections, Syphilis.

17. B. Yellow fever

Yellow fever is a live vaccination and is therefore not recommended in pregnancy. Other live vaccinations not recommended include MMR, oral typhoid, and oral polio. Hepatitis A and B vaccinations are composed of viral antigens, and tetanus vaccination is a toxoid.

Collins S et al., *Oxford Handbook of Obstetrics and Gynaecology*, Second Edition, Oxford University Press, 2008, Chapter 4, Infectious diseases in pregnancy, Vaccination and travel.

18. A. Sodium valproate

Sodium valproate or lamotrigine is the first-line choice for generalized epilepsy. Second-line drugs include levetiracetam or topiramate.

Manji H et al., *Oxford Handbook of Neurology*, Oxford University Press, 2007, Chapter 4, Neurological disorders.

19. B. Carbamazepine

Carbamazepine is the usual first-line antileptic medication for focal seizures. Lamotrigine and valproate would also be considered as first-line choices. Levetiracetam and topiramate would be considered as second-line alternatives.

Manji H et al., *Oxford Handbook of Neurology*, Oxford University Press, 2007, Chapter 4, Neurological disorders.

20. E. Goodpasture's disease with neurological complications

The mechanisms by which intravenous immunoglobulin (IVIg) plasma exchange work are unclear but theories include anti-idiotypic antibodies, maximal saturation, and blockade of Fc receptors on macrophages or via the modulation of pro-inflammatory cytokines. IVIg has a role in numerous neurological disorders, but plasma exchange is the treatment of choice for Goodpasture's disease where the antibody itself is pathogenic causing the vasculitis.

Manji H et al., *Oxford Handbook of Neurology*, Oxford University Press, 2007, Chapter 4, Neurological disorders.

21. A. Add a long-acting beta2 agonist inhaler (salmeterol)

It is important to know the stepwise management of chronic asthma in MRCP Part 1.

Longmore M et al., *Oxford Handbook of Clinical Medicine*, Eighth Edition, Oxford University Press, 2010, Chapter 4, Chest medicine, Management of chronic asthma.

22. D. Nicorandil

Nicorandil is recognized as a rare cause of anal ulceration and fissuring, and the condition usually settles down rapidly after the medication is discontinued. Switching or discontinuation of nicorandil should only take place on the advice of a cardiologist.

For full list of side effects associated with Nicorandil. https://www.medicines.org.uk/emc/medicine/28327.

23. B. Sunitinib

A recent MHRA alert drew attention to case reports of osteonecrosis of the jaw (ONJ) in conjunction with use of sunitinib and bevacizumab. Patients in these case reports were also in many cases taking bisphosphonates or had other risk factors such as recent radiotherapy treatment. As both drugs inhibit osteogenesis, however, there may well be a pathophysiological reason why ONJ may occur in conjunction with their use. Risk factors for ONJ include: bisphosphonates; malignant disease; use of corticosteroids; chemotherapy; radiotherapy; poor oral hygiene; smoking; and dental or orofacial surgical procedures.

Gov.uk, Bevacizumab and sunitinib: risk of osteonecrosis of the jaw. http://www.mhra.gov.uk/Safetyinformation/DrugSafetyUPDAte/CON105745.

24. C. Hydroxycobalamin

Exposure to polyurethane foam combustion products is suggestive of possible cyanide poisoning, and the patient's symptoms are also supportive of this underlying diagnosis. Five grams of hydroxycobalamin infused over 15–30 minutes is one possible treatment for cyanide poisoning. Other options include disodium EDTA for more severe symptoms, sodium nitrite, and sodium thiosulphate. Any possible skin contamination requires washing with soap and water as cyanide may be absorbed through the skin, and mouth-to-mouth resuscitation should not be attempted.

Ramrakha PS et al., *Oxford Handbook of Acute Medicine*, Third Edition, Oxford University Press, 2010, Chapter 14, Drug overdoses, Cyanide.

25. B. Apomorphine

Selegiline is a MAO-B inhibitor, and pergolide is an ergot-derived dopamine agonist. Whilst pergolide is potentially useful in on/off phenomena, the fact that it is ergot-derived means that it is not a first-choice agent. Apomorphine in contrast is particularly useful in on/off phenomena, although it is delivered subcutaneously. Providers have developed a number of portable pump options to ease delivery.

emc+, Apomorphine 10mg/ml solution for injection. http://www.medicines.org.uk/EMC/medicine/21983/SPC/Apomorphine%2010mg%20ml%20solution%20for%20injection/.

26. B. Bicarbonate

In this situation the default treatment is correction of acidosis, with sodium bicarbonate IV, either given as repeated boluses or as an IV infusion with the aim of targeting a pH of 7.5–7.55. If VT persists then lignocaine can be added. Some case series have also suggested that IV magnesium may be of value in reversing VT.

Wyatt J et al., *Oxford Handbook of Emergency Medicine*, Fourth Edition, Oxford University Press, 2012, Chapter 4, Toxicology, Tricyclic antidepressant poisoning.

27. B. Diuretic

Hypercalcaemia is a side effect of thiazide diuretics. Furosemide increases calcium excretion while thiazides decrease it. It is of interest that post-menopausal women on thiazides have a lower incidence of osteoporosis as the negative calcium balance that is associated with the menopause may be reduced with concomitant thiazide therapy.

Ramrakha PS et al., *Oxford Handbook of Acute Medicine*, Third Edition, Oxford University Press, Chapter 9, Endocrine emergencies, Hypercalcaemia.

28. B. Fludrocortisone

All the replacement therapies listed are appropriate for an individual with hypopituitarism with the exception of fludrocortisone, the secretion of which is not under the control of the pituitary but rather the renin-angiotensin system.

Longmore M et al., *Oxford Handbook of Clinical Medicine*, Eighth Edition, Oxford University Press, 2010, Chapter 5, Endocrinology, Hypopituitarism.

29. D. Withhold methotrexate and give folinic acid

This lady has significant sepsis in the context of pancytopenia, which is likely to be related to methotrexate toxicity. Methotrexate is a folic acid antagonist with immunosuppressive and cytotoxic actions. It is used at relatively low doses in psoriasis, inflammatory arthritis, and Crohn's disease, and at higher doses in cancer chemotherapy. Folic acid is often co-prescribed with the aim of reducing the risk of marrow toxicity. The optimal dose of folic acid is debated, as its effects on the efficacy of methotrexate are not clear. Marrow toxicity from methotrexate may occur abruptly during treatment. Sometimes, no cause is apparent.

However, factors to explore include the possibility of drug interaction: some drugs increase plasma levels of methotrexate (e.g. non-steroidal anti-inflammatory drugs), and concurrent use of another folate antagonist (e.g. trimethoprim) increases the risk of toxicity. Adherence to the prescribed dose should be checked (note that it is usually prescribed once weekly); also, bear in mind that 2.5 mg methotrexate tablets are usually dispensed for low-dose regimes, yet 10 mg tablets also exist. Treatment of probable marrow toxicity complicated by sepsis, as in the case described, includes withholding methotrexate and the administration of intravenous folinic acid.

Maxtrex [methotrexate] tablets 2.5 mg, Summary of Product Characteristics, Pharmacia, 2008. http://www.medicines.org.uk/EMC/medicine/6003/SPC/Maxtrex+Tablets+2.5+mg/.

30. A. 2,3-dimercaptopropanesulphonate (DMPS)

DMPS (or the similar chelating agent DMSA) is the treatment of choice for acute severe arsenic toxicity. Dicobalt edetate is used for cyanide poisoning. Desferrioxamine is used for treatment of iron (and aluminium) toxicity. Pralidoxime is an acetylcholinesterase reactivator and is used following organophosphorus poisoning.

Warrell DA et al., *Oxford Textbook of Medicine*, Fifth Edition, Oxford University Press, 2010, Section 9.1, Poisoning by drugs and chemicals.

31. C. Fluconazole and simvastatin

Fluconazole decreases the metabolism of HMG-CoA reductase inhibitors and in the presence of renal impairment the risk of developing rhabdomyolysis increases even more. If ciprofloxacin is used in combination with fluconazole, which is known to increase the QT interval, the risk of cardiac arrhythmias increases. No significant interactions have been noted for the rest of the combinations.

British National Formulary. https://www.evidence.nhs.uk/formulary/bnf/current/5-infections/52-antifungal-drugs/521-triazole-antifungals/fluconazole.

32. C. Ethambutol

Ethambutol may cause a dose-related optic neuritis. This may manifest as reduced colour vision, loss of visual acuity, central scotoma or peripheral field defect. Isoniazid may lead to a peripheral neuropathy, which can usually be prevented by giving pyridoxine. Rifampicin and isoniazid may uncommonly cause a hepatitis.

Warrell DA et al., *Oxford Textbook of Medicine*, Fifth Edition, Oxford University Press, 2010, Section 7.6.25, Tuberculosis.

33. A. Rivaroxaban

Ribaroxaban is a direct factor Xa inhibitor, while dabigatran is a direct thrombin inhibitor. Enoxaparin is a low molecular weight heparin, which binds and potentiates the inhibitory activity of antithrombin III on factor Xa. Clopidogrel is an antiplatelet agent which acts via inhibition of the P2Y12 receptor.

Ahrens I, Lip GY, Peter K, New oral anticoagulant drugs in cardiovascular disease, *Thrombosis and Haemostasis* 2010;104(1):49–60.

34. A. *RYR1*

Malignant hyperthermia shows some genetic heterogeneity, but the majority of mutations described are within the RYR1 gene, which codes for the ryanodine receptor isoform 1. Common triggering agents to malignant hyperthermia include volatile anaesthetic agents (e.g. halothane, sevoflurane) and depolarizing muscle paralysing drugs such as succinylcholine.

Litman RS, Rosenberg H, Malignant hyperthermia: update on susceptibility testing, *Journal of the American Medical Association* 2005; 293(23):2918–2924.

35. B. Bromocriptine

This patient has neuroleptic malignant syndrome as evidenced by the recent prescription of haloperidol and symptoms consistent with the disorder. Treatment has centred around use of either dopamine agonists such as bromocriptine and drugs that uncouple muscle metabolism such as dantrolene. Randomized controlled trial evidence is sparse, but evidence suggests that the time course of symptoms and prognosis is improved more with the use of dopamine agonists compared to dantrolene. As such bromocriptine is the treatment of choice. Patients may of course also require benzodiazepines if they are particularly agitated.

emc+, Parlodel 5mg Capsules. http://www.medicines.org.uk/emc/medicine/2373/SPC/Parlodel+5mg+Capsules/.

36. B. Imatinib

Imatinib is an inhibitor of the bcr-abl fusion tyrosine kinase, constitutively activated by the Philadelphia translocation in CML. Sunitinib is also a tyrosine kinase inhibitor, used predominantly for treatment of renal cell carcinoma. Gemtuzumab is a monoclonal antibody to CD33 used in the treatment of AML. Rituximab is a monoclonal antibody to the B-cell marker CD20, primarily for the treatment of non-Hodgkin's lymphoma. Cetuximab is a monoclonal antibody to VEGF-A, which is licensed for use in colorectal cancer and non-small cell lung cancer.

Marin D, Current status of imatinib as frontline therapy for chronic myeloid leukemia, *Seminars in Hematology* 2010;47(4):312–318.

37. E. Continue paracetamol and add codeine

In this situation, the WHO analgesic ladder should be used to manage this gentleman's pain. He has tried step 1, and should therefore move to step 2 (Figure 4.1). This involves adding a weak opioid to his existing paracetamol. Given that he has advanced cancer he should have regular reviews regarding his pain, and may need further increases in the level of analgesia.

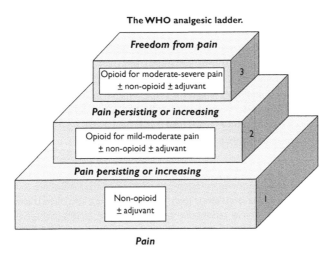

Figure 4.1 WHO analgesic ladder

Adapted from *World Health Organization*, WHO's cancer pain ladder for adults, http://www.who.int/cancer/palliative/painladder/en/ (accessed January 2016).

Watson M et al., *Oxford Handbook of Palliative Care*, Second Edition, Oxford University Press, 2009, Chapter 6a, The management of pain: The principles of pain management, Step 2 analgesics.

38. C. Dipyridamole

Dipyridamole inhibits the cellular uptake of adenosine, potentiating its cardiac effects of AV block, and may even precipitate asystole. As such, adenosine should be used with caution or avoided in patients taking dipyridamole.

Rang HP, Dale MM, *Pharmacology*, Churchill Livingstone, 2007.

39. B. Xanthine oxidase inhibitor

Allopurinol is a xanthine oxidase inhibitor. This enzyme is part of the pathway that forms uric acid. Inhibition of this pathway reduces uric acid levels. This drug is often given to patients as prophylaxis when they have a high risk of developing tumour lysis syndrome. Statins are commonly used HMG co-A reductase inhibitors and are used to reduce cholesterol. An example of a drug that suppresses T cell activity is the biologic abatacept An example of a medication that suppresses B cells is the biologic rituximab. Uricosuric drugs act by increasing uric acid excretion in the urine. The most commonly used uricosuric drug is probenacid.

BNF, Section 10.1.4, Gout and cytotoxic-induced hyperuricaemia, Subsection: Long-term control of gout. https://www.evidence.nhs.uk/formulary/bnf/current/10-musculoskeletal-and-joint-diseases/ 101-drugs-used-in-rheumatic-diseases-and-gout/1014-gout-and-cytotoxic-induced-hyperuricaemia/ long-term-control-of-gout.

40. C. Metaclopramide

Metaclopramide is a pro-kinetic agent, and as such is known to reduce absorption of paracetamol. This may have accounted for the decreased pain-relieving effects of this man's regular medication. In contrast, propantheline leads to reduced gastric emptying and as such leads to increased paracetamol absorption. Despite the fact that omeprazole induces CYP1A2, no increase in paracetamol toxicity due to NAPQI formation is seen.

Drug and health products, Health Canada, http://www.hc-sc.gc.ca/dhp-mps/medeff/advisories-avis/ index-eng.php.

41. B. TNF antagonist

Adalimumab binds directly to TNF and blocks its biological action by preventing it interacting with the p55 and p75 cell surface TNF receptors. It therefore modulates a range of downstream biological responses which are modulated by TNF. This mode of action is subtly different from other biologicals such as etanercept which competitively inhibit the action of TNF by binding to the TNF receptor itself. Like the TNF receptor antagonists, reactivation of tuberculosis is a recognized adverse event.

emc+, Humira Pre-filled Pen, Pre-filled Syringe and Vial. http://www.medicines.org.uk/emc/medicine/ 21201/SPC/Humira+Pen+and+Syringe/.

42. C. Infliximab

Infliximab is approved by NICE for use in severe psoriasis when the PASI score is >20, and the dermatology quality of life index is greather than 18. Patients must also have trialed conventional immunomodulatory therapy such as ciclosporin or methotrexate. In this case, given the patient has severe disease despite PUVA and ciclosporin, infliximab is the next most logical step. NICE does however stipulate a 10-week limit to treatment unless there is a >75% improvement in the PASI score, or a >50% improvement with a significant improvement in quality of life.

Psoriasis: assessment and management, NICE Guidelines (CG 153) Published October 2012

43. E. Cyclizine

Cyclizine is an antihistamine anti-emetic and is therefore not associated with risk of acute dystonia. Both prochlorperazine (stemetil) and metaclopramide (maxolon) are dopamine antagonists and their use should be avoided in young women. Hyoscine is commonly used in travel sickness pills and is an anti-muscarinic agent. 5-HT antagonists such as ondansetron are also relatively free of adverse events.

Flake ZA et al., Practical selection of antiemetics, *American Family Physician* 2004;1;69(5):1169–1174. http://www.aafp.org/afp/2004/0301/p1169.html.

44. A. Insulin aspart

Insulin pump therapy requires short-acting insulin, and as such insulin aspart is the most appropriate answer. Insulin lispro is also commonly used. Insulin glulisine may be used in pump therapy, but there are thought to be only minor differences between aspart, lispro, and glulisine with respect to clinical outcomes, and the evidence base is significantly larger currently for aspart use in pumps. Studies of subcutaneous insulin pumps used in pregnancy suggest that there is reduced weight gain and less hypo and hyperglycaemia versus patients taking a traditional basal bolus regimen.

Insulin aspart summary of product characteristics. http://www.medicines.org.uk/EMC/medicine/25033/SPC/NovoRapid+100+U+ml+in+a+vial%2c+NovoRapid+Penfill+100+U+ml%2c+NovoRapid+Flex Pen+100+U+ml%2c+NovoRapid+FlexTouch+100+U+ml/.

45. A. Akthisia

Akathisia is a typical side effect associated with the use of olanzapine. Other side effects are exacerbation of Parkinson's disease, neutropaenia, hyperprolactinaemia, increased appetite, and rhabdomyolysis.

Collier J et al., *Oxford Handbook of Clinical Specialties*, Eighth Edition, Oxford University Press, 2009, Chapter 4, Psychiatry, Schizophrenia: management.

46. E. Peripheral oedema without heart failure

Pioglitazone is a PPAR-gamma agonist which leads to up-regulation of a number of genes associated with lipid metabolism, leading to a fall in free fatty acids and a reduction in central fat, and an increase in peripheral fat. Pioglitazone is also associated with a small fall in blood pressure of around 5/3 mmHg and positive changes in HDL cholesterol, although it is associated with a small rise in LDL. Peripheral oedema is common (in around 10% of patients), and heart failure is also reported. It is also thought that changes in marrow fat lead to increased risk of osteoporosis.

emc+, Actos tables. http://www.medicines.org.uk/emc/medicine/4236.

47. A. Ecstasy overdose

This patient is hyperpyrexial with evidence of rhabdomyolysis as evidenced by the raised CK. Put together with the dilated pupils and increased tone, this is consistent with an ecstasy overdose. Management is on the HDU/ITU, specifically aimed at reducing the hyperpyrexia, and taking control of fluid balance. Early recognition of the symptoms and signs of ecstasy overdose is crucial with respect to reducing mortality.

Kaye S et al., Methylenedioxymethamphetamine (MDMA)-related fatalities in Australia: demographics, circumstances, toxicology and major organ pathology, *Drug and Alcohol Dependence* 2009;104:251–261. http://www.sciencedirect.com/science?_ob=ArticleURL&_udi=B6T63-4WS2239-2&_user=10&_coverDate=10%2F01%2F2009&_rdoc=1&_fmt=high&_orig=search&_origin=search&_sort=d&_docanchor=&view=c&_searchStrId=1538876897&_rerunOrigin=scholar.google&_acct=C000050221&_vers.

48. C. PPAR-alpha agonist

Fibrates are PPAR-alpha agonists. Activation of this particular nuclear receptor leads to up-regulation of a number of genes which deal with lipid handling, including up-regulation of lipoprotein lipase, which increases lipolysis and the elimination of triglyceride-rich particles from plasma. PPAR-gamma agonists are the glitazones, which up-regulate genes that deal with insulin resistance in fat, leading to an increase in subcutaneous fat storage and a decrease in central fat. The statins of course are HMG-coA reductase inhibitors. With respect to fibrates, outcome studies have been slightly disappointing with respect to additive effects on CV risk reduction compared to statins alone. One recent study, the ACCORD study, did show a trend to benefit, combined with statins in those patients with type 2 diabetes who have low HDL and raised triglycerides.

Staels B et al., Cardiovascular drugs: mechanism of action of fibrates on lipid and lipoprotein Metabolism, *Circulation* 1998;98:2088–2093.

49. B. Anti-platelet agent

Sarpogrelate is a 5HT-2B receptor antagonist, which interferes with platelet aggregation. It is licensed in a number of countries in Asia such as Japan and Korea, where it is used as an alternative to aspirin therapy. 5HT-2A and 2C receptor antagonists are centrally acting, and are used as atypical anti-psychotics. 5HT-3 antagonists are used as anti-emetics, the best example of which is ondansetron. Finally, amongst 5-HT1 receptors, 1B and 1D receptor agonists are used in the treatment of migraine, the best example of which is zomatriptan. Buspirone is a 1A receptor agonist, used as an anxiolytic antidepressant.

Harvey R, Champe P (eds), *Lippincott Illustrated Reviews: Pharmacology*, Fourth Edition, Lippincott Williams & Wilkins, 2009.

50. D. Pravastatin

A number of agents for immunosuppression, including ciclosporin, tacrolimus, and sirolimus, are metabolized by CYP3A4, and as such simvastatin and atorvastatin coadministration can lead to significant changes in levels of these drugs. Given their narrow therapeutic range, even a small change in levels can lead to inadequate immunosuppression or toxicity. Pravastatin is not signficantly metabolized by CYP3A4, and as such is a reasonable choice. Rosuvastatin is only 10% metabolized by CYP450, and mainly by CYP2C9. Both are alternatives in patients taking immunosuppressive medication. Pravastatin prescribing information, http://www.medicines.org.uk/emc/medicine/25734.

51. C. Luminosities within the visual fields

Ivabradine is an inhibitor of the cardiac 'funny' channels, which are responsible for diastolic depolarization of the sinus node. Blockade of these channels results in bradycardia and therefore the medication is used as a treatment for rate-dependent angina. It is a second-line therapy for patients who are unable to take beta-blockade. The commonest reported adverse event is patients seeing luminosities within their visual field and this is caused because of cross reactivity with the Ih channels present within the retina.

emc+, Procoralan. http://www.medicines.org.uk/emc/medicine/17188/SPC/Procoralan/.

52. A. Three days

Denosumab is an IgG monoclonal antibody and a rank ligand inhibitor. Rank ligand is responsible for driving pre-osteoclast to osteoclast maturation, and up-regulating osteoclast activity. Inhibiting this therefore leads to an 85% fall in carboxy-terminal collagen crosslinks by day 3, a marker of bone resorption. The reduction is around 40% by the time denosumab is re-dosed at month 6. The antibody is used in patients who are unable to tolerate bisphosphonate therapy.

emc+, Prolia. http://www.medicines.org.uk/EMC/medicine/23127/SPC/Prolia/.

53. B. Diarrhoea

Strontium ranelate substitutes calcium ions in bone and is associated with a measured increase of up to 15% in BMD at the lumbar spine, and up to 6% at the hip, although BMD increases measured by DEXA are overestimated because of differences between strontium and calcium in their level of DEXA absorption. Strontium has been shown in animal models to be associated with an increase in trabecular bone formation. The commonest reported adverse events in the strontium ranelate study programme included nausea and diarrhoea.

emc+, Protelos: undesirable effects. http://www.medicines.org.uk/emc/medicine/ 15410#UNDESIRABLE_EFFECTS.

54. E. Hyperglycaemia

Bendroflumethiazide acts at the site of the thiazide-sensitive sodium/chloride transporter in the distal convoluted tubule. This results in increased sodium excretion; distally, this promotes overactivity of the aldosterone-sensitive transporter which leads to hypokalaemia. Other effects of thiazides include hypercalcaemia and hyperuricaemia. A meta-analysis of beta-blocker and thiazide combined therapy has demonstrated an increased risk of incident diabetes, and at an individual patient level, thiazide use may be associated with a worsening in blood glucose control.

emc+, Aprinox / Bendroflumethiazide 2.5 and 5mg Tablets. http://www.medicines.org.uk/emc/ document.aspx?documentId=13049.

55. C. Bradykinin

Accumulation of bradykinin in response to angiotensin-converting enzyme inhibition is thought to be responsible for the cough associated with therapy. Of course, because angiotensin receptor blockers only block the site of action of angiotensin 2, they do not lead to bradykinin inhibition and do not cause the cough. Whilst ACE inhibitors may be associated with a slightly worse side effect profile in respect of the cough, the incidence of angioedema is similar between classes, and efficacy data, if anything, suggest a slightly lower frequency of ischaemic cardiovascular events associated with ACE inhibitor use.

emc+, Ramipril 10mg Capsules. http://www.medicines.org.uk/EMC/medicine/24148/SPC/ Ramipril+10mg+Capsules/.

56. E. High-dose inhaled corticosteroids and long-acting beta-2 agonist therapy

The TORCH study demonstrated the positive impact on exacerbation frequency of high-dose inhaled corticosteroid and long-acting beta agonist therapy. This was however at the expense of increased risk of episodes of pneumonia. With respect to mortality, the TORCH study narrowly missed its mortality endpoint, but you could conclude that the study showed a strong trend towards mortality benefit.

Peter MA et al., on behalf of the TORCH investigators, Salmeterol and fluticasone propionate and survival in chronic obstructive pulmonary disease, *New England Journal of Medicine* 2007;356:775–789.

57. C. Proximal convoluted tubule

Acetazolamide is a carbonic anhydrase inhibitor which leads to increased excretion of sodium and bicarbonate and is a weak diuretic. In practice its major use is in the treatment of glaucoma to reduce intra-ocular pressure, and in ophthalmic surgery. It is also used in the treatment of altitude sickness when access to medical services or the chance to descend may be delayed. A major side-effect of acetazolamide therapy is a large increase in symptoms of gastro-oesophageal reflux disease, which may limit its use beyond a few days for many patients.

emc+, Acetazolamide: undersirable effects. http://www.medicines.org.uk/emc/medicine/22217/SPC/DIAMOX+Tablets+250mg/#UNDESIRABLE_EFFECTS.

58. C. Xa

Rivaroxaban is a factor Xa inhibitor that is currently licensed for prophylaxis against venous thromboembolism in patients undergoing orthopaedic surgery. In patients undergoing major procedures such as hip replacement, prophylaxis for up to five weeks is recommended, with two weeks the recommended limit for more minor surgery. Increases in transaminases are commonly seen with rivaroxaban, although more serious hepatic dysfunction and a rise in amylase are much rarer. The major advantage of factor Xa inhibitors is that they do not require INR monitoring.

emc+, Xarelto 10 mg film-coated tablets. http://www.medicines.org.uk/emc/medicine/21265.

59. D. NPC1L1 inhibitor

Ezetimibe is an inhibitor of the Niemann-Pick C1-Like1 (NPC1L1) transporter which is the intestinal transporter that is responsible for absorption of cholesterol and plant sterols. By inhibiting it, ezetimibe achieves a reduction in LDL cholesterol of around 25%. Whilst the magnitude of cholesterol reduction is not as great as that of a statin in monotherapy, combinations of statin and ezetimibe are also available. Abdominal pain, diarrhoea, and flatulence are the most commonly reported adverse events associated with ezetimibe therapy.

emc+, Exetrol: Pharmacodynamic properties. http://www.medicines.org.uk/EMC/medicine/12091/SPC/Ezetrol+10mg+Tablets/#PHARMACODYNAMIC_PROPS.

60. D. Beta-2 partial agonist

Salmeterol is a partial beta-2 agonist which has a long half-life, and is therefore given twice a day in conjunction with inhaled corticosteroids. It is recommended as add-in to medium-dose inhaled corticosteroids by the BTS guidelines as an alternative to uptitration of inhaled steroid dose. Because it is a high-affinity partial agonist, there is a theoretical risk that excess use may reduce the effectiveness of salbutamol therapy. It is also associated with increased risk of atrial tachycardias when used in patients with COPD.

emc+, Serevent Evohaler. http://www.medicines.org.uk/EMC/medicine/17201/SPC/Serevent%20 Evohaler/.

61. D. Tacrolimus

Both sirolimus and tacrolimus are associated with increased risk of diabetes mellitus. This is thought to be related to mitochondrial dysfunction which leads to increased insulin resistance. Of the two, however, the risk is higher with tacrolimus and as such transplant immunosuppression regimes in patients with a history of diabetes mellitus or cardiovascular disease have become largely tacrolimus free. That being said, patients should be encouraged to work hard with respect to weight control, and cardiovascular risk factors such as hypertension and dyslipidaemia should be managed aggressively.

Woordward RS et al., Incidence and cost of new onset diabetes mellitus among U.S. wait-listed and transplanted renal allograft recipients, *American Journal of Transplantation* 2003;3:590–598. http://onlinelibrary.wiley.com/doi/10.1034/j.1600-6143.2003.00082.x/full.

emc+, Tacrolimus: undesirable effects. http://www.medicines.org.uk/emc/medicine/11102#UNDESIRABLE_EFFECTS.

62. D. Renin antagonist

Aliskiren binds to the s3b pocket of renin, which blocks renin activity leading to blockade of conversion of angiotensinogen to angiotensin 1 and angiotensin 1 to angiotensin 2. It also leads to a 50–80% reduction in plasma renin activity. Early studies suggest that it may be more effective than ACE inhibition in the management of diabetic renal disease, and that it may be better than ACE inhibitors with respect to reducing cyst formation in autosomal dominant polycystic kidney disease. It is, however, still associated with angioedema.

emc+, Rasilez 150mg film-coated tablets. http://www.medicines.org.uk/emc/document. aspx?documentId=20049.

63. A. G-protein-coupled receptor

The parathyroid hormone receptor is a G-protein-coupled receptor. They are integral membrane receptors that have seven membrane spanning domains. There are thought to be around 800 G-protein-coupled receptors so far identified. These include the parathyroid hormone receptor, mutations of which lead to hypoparathyroidism because of parathyroid hormone resistance. Other examples of G-protein-coupled receptors include rhodopsin, and receptors which are thought to account for the action of other hormones, such as GLP-1, which is thought to act in part via the GPR 119 receptor.

Cafiero A, Drug–receptor interactions, Merck Manual.

64. D. 50

One hundred patients treated with the new treatment have a 4% hypertension rate, versus 2% for those treated with the leading alternative. This means that the number needed to harm with respect to hypertension is $100/(4-2) = 50$. In other words, for every 50 patients treated with the new treatment versus the old one, one patient would suffer a hypertension-related adverse event. Whether this is acceptable of course depends upon the efficacy profile of the agent versus the traditional comparator.

Calculating and using NNTS, Bandolier Extra 2003; February. http://www.medicine.ox.ac.uk/bandolier/ Extraforbando/NNTextra.pdf.

65. C. Serious adverse event, should be reported immediately to the sponsor

A serious adverse event (SAE) in human drug trials is defined as any untoward medical occurrence that (at any dose) results in death, is life-threatening, requires inpatient hospitalization or prolongation of existing hospitalization, results in persistent or significant disability/incapacity, or is a congenital anomaly/birth defect. In this context, the myocardial infarction that your patient has suffered is consistent with a serious adverse event. Regulatory timelines are very tight, and clinical trialists should report SAEs as soon as possible to representatives of the study sponsor.

European Medicines Agency, ICH topic E 2 A: Clinical safety data management: definitions and standards for expedited reporting, Step 5, EMEA, 1995. http://www.ema.europa.eu/docs/en_GB/ document_library/Scientific_guideline/2009/09/WC500002749.pdf.

66. C. Competitive antagonist of alcohol dehydrogenase

Fomepizole, or 4-methyl pyrazole, is a competitive antagonist of alcohol dehydrogenase. The major advantage over ethanol in treating overdose of methanol or ethylene glycol is that it is not sedative. By interfering with the action of alcohol dehydrogenase on ethylene glycol, fomepizole leads to a reduction in the formation of glycolate and oxalate, the products of metabolism responsible for renal failure post ethylene glycol overdose. With respect to methanol, fomepizole interferes with the production of formaldehyde and thence formic acid.

Brent J, Fomepizole for ethylene glycol and methanol poisoning, *New England Journal of Medicine* 2009;360:2216–2223. http://www.nejm.org/doi/full/10.1056/NEJMct0806112.

67. A. Ciprofloxacin

CYP 1A2 is the enzyme responsible for metabolism of both ciprofloxacin and theophylline. Ciprofloxacin is a significant inhibitor of 1A2, which can lead to accumulation of toxic levels of theophylline. This can lead an to increased risk of nausea and vomiting, and a risk of tachyarrhythmias. Whilst the macrolides erythromycin and clarithromycin are predominantly 3A4 inhibitors, they are also associated with an increase in theophylline levels and risk of toxicity. As such, the most appropriate choice for antibiotic therapy is likely to be co-amoxiclav.

Paulsen O et al., The interaction of erythromycin with theophylline, *European Journal of Clinical Pharmacology* 1987;32(5):493–498. http://www.ncbi.nlm.nih.gov/pubmed/3622597.

68. B. Oxidation

Phase 1 and phase 2 reactions are both involved in hepatic drug metabolism. Phase 1 reactions include oxidation, reduction, and hydrolysis, and are designed essentially to make drugs more polar to assist in their elimination. These processes are mediated by CYP450 enzymes. Phase 2 reactions involve either conjugation with glutathione, sulphonation, acetylation, or glucuronidation as typical examples. CYP450/Phase 1 reactions are usually most impacted by drug–drug interactions.

Good introduction to drug reactions: https://en.wikipedia.org/wiki/Drug_metabolism.

69. C. Functional class 3 PAH without significant interstitial lung disease

Bosentan is an endothelin receptor antagonist and is one of a class of therapies used in the treatment of pulmonary hypertension. It is indicated in the treatment of functional class 3 PAH but can only be used in scleroderma in the absence of interstitial lung disease. There is significant debate about sequencing of therapies in PAH and a number of combination studies are underway. There is no restriction on sequencing of endothelin receptor-based therapies with respect to before or after PDE5 inhibitors or prostaglandin.

2015 ESC/ERS Guidelines for the diagnosis and treatment of pulmonary hypertension. *European Heart Journal.* doi:10.1093/eurheartj/ehv317.

70. B. Metaclopramide

Dopamine antagonist anti-emetics are associated with an increased risk of acute dystonic reactions, particularly in young women. The two commonest dopamine antagonist anti-emetics used are either prochlorperazine, or metaclopramide, hence metaclopramide listed here is most likely to be the cause of her symptoms. Treatment of acute dystonia is with anticholinergics. For this patient group, domperidone or cyclizine are the usual first-line therapies.

Van Harten P et al., Acute dystonia induced by drug treatment, *British Medical Journal* 1999;319:623–626. http://www.ncbi.nlm.nih.gov/pmc/articles/PMC1116493/.

71. A. Lipoprotein lipase activator

Fibrates are PPAR-alpha activators, leading to upregulation of lipid-handling enzymes which include lipoprotein lipase, and consequent decrease in triglycerides and increase in HDL. Ezetimibe selectively inhibits the absorption of cholesterol and selected plant sterols from the border of the small intestine. It does this by inhibiting the NPC1L1 transporter. Statins are inhibitors of HMG-CoA reductase.

emd+, Exetrol: pharmacodynamics properties. http://www.medicines.org.uk/emc/medicine/
12091#PHARMACODYNAMIC_PROPS.

72. B. Atenolol

The atypical antipsychotic, olanzapine, is not associated with worsening psoriasis; the commonly
used mood stabilizer, lithium, is, however. Atenolol and other beta-blockers are associated with
worsening of psoriasis. It is believed that this is caused by decreased intra-epidermal cyclic AMP
production inducing epidermal hyperproliferation. Ciclosporin may be used as systemic treatment
for severe psoriasis. Its dermatological complications include hypertrichosis and an increased
incidence of skin tumours. Paracetamol does not affect the rash of psoriasis. Amiodarone is often
associated with a photosensitive rash but does not affect psoriasis.

Schön MP, Boehncke WH, Psoriasis (Review), *New England Journal of Medicine* 2005;352:1899–1912.
http://www.nejm.org/doi/pdf/10.1056/NEJMra041320.

73. B. Clarithromycin

Ciclosporin is metabolized by CYP 3A4, for this reason any patient co-prescribed a 3A4 inhibitor
is likely to experience a significant increase in their ciclosporin levels, putting them at risk of
nephrotoxicity. The macrolide antibiotics are one group metabolized by 3A4, and are significant
inhibitors of the enzyme. Both erythromycin and clarithromycin should not be used in combination
with ciclosporin. Azithromycin does not share the same level of 3A4 inhibition. Other important
3A4 inhibitors include the azole anti-fungal agents, verapamil, diltiazem, and grapefruit juice. In this
situation, if the patient is not allergic to penicillins, then amoxicillin would be the logical first-choice
antibiotic.

emc+, Neoral Soft Gelatin Capsules. http://www.medicines.org.uk/EMC/medicine/1307/SPC/Neoral+
Soft+Gelatin+Capsules%2c+Neoral+Oral+Solution/.

74. D. Ramipril

Medications are frequently implicated in the development of gynaecomastia, particularly drugs
used in the management of hypertension and cardiac failure. Of the drugs listed, ramipril (an ACE
inhibitor) is the one associated strongly with development of gynaecomastia; the remainder are
not. The mechanism by which ACE inhibitors cause gynaecomastia is not entirely clear. Digoxin
has some oestrogen-like properties and hence causes gynaecomastia. Spironolactone causes
gynaecomastia because it is associated with the displacement of androgen from androgen receptors
and sex hormone-binding globulin, increased metabolic clearance of testosterone, and higher
oestradiol production. A well-known useful acronym for drugs associated with gynaecomastia is
MADRAS (Marijuana, ACE inhibitors, Digoxin, Ranitidine, Alcohol, and Spironolactone).

Prisant LM, Chin E, Gynecomastia and hypertension, *Journal of Clinical Hypertension* (Greenwich)
2005;7:245–248.

75. C. Factor Xa inhibitor

Rivaroxaban is one of a new class of oral anti-coagulants, which appear to offer a similar level of
efficacy to warfarin, but without the need for therapeutic monitoring. Currently, they are licensed
for the prophylaxis of venous thromboembolism in patients undergoing joint replacement therapy.
They act as direct factor Xa inhibitors, blocking the clotting cascade and inhibiting the formation
of thrombin. Common adverse events include elevated liver enzymes, although serious hepatic
dysfunction is rarer. Nausea is also commonly reported.

emc+, Rivaroxaban: pharmacodynamics properties. http://www.medicines.org.uk/emc/medicine/
21265#PHARMACODYNAMIC_PROPS.

76. A. It is converted to a pyrimidine analogue

Capecitabine is an oral precursor for 5-fluorouracil, which is a pyrimidine analogue that is a non-competitive antagonist of thymidylate synthase, meaning that it interferes with the synthesis of DNA. Given that cancer cells undergo rapid turnover, they are particularly affected by 5-FU administration. Data comparing capecitabine to 5-FU given intravenously suggests there is little difference between the two in terms of efficacy, and oral versus intravenous administration brings tolerability advantages. Gastrointestinal disorders, vomiting, diarrhoea, anorexia, and stomatitis are the most commonly reported adverse events.

emc+, Xeloda 150mg and 500mg Film-coated Tablets. http://www.medicines.org.uk/emc/medicine/ 4619.

77. D. Phase 3 study

Phase 1 studies are the first-time-in-man studies, to determine whether an agent is safe enough to be progressed further. They are small and involve testing single and multiple doses of a new drug in healthy volunteers. Phase 2 studies are designed to give information about the likely therapeutic dose in patients who have a particular disease. The dose that is deemed most effective, normally after examination of surrogate markers, is the one that is carried into phase 3, a group of confirmatory studies designed to compare the effect of a drug in a larger number of patients, versus the usual standard of care. Phase 4 studies may be used to make marketing claims, or provide other data, such as real-life epidemiology studies. In the case of reimbursement agencies, such as NICE or the SMC, the highest quality of phase 3 randomized control trial evidence is usually required.

Clinicaltrials.gov, Learn about clinical trials. http://clinicaltrials.gov/ct2/info/understand.

78. A. Buprenorphine

Buprenorphine is a partial opiate agonist. This means that at full receptor occupancy, it still does not achieve the same physiological effect as a full opiate agonist such as morphine. It has slowly reversible binding with opioid mu receptors, which means it can minimize the need for opioid-addicted patients to use drugs for a prolonged period of time. Studies suggest that it limits positive mood changes, good feelings, and respiratory depression, which occur in conjunction with opiate abuse. Naloxone is an opiate receptor antagonist, which may be given in combination with buprenorphine as a combination tablet. The reason for this is that it limits the ability of addicts to make a liquid from the pills and inject them to gain a high. Flumazenil is a benzodiazepine receptor antagonist.

emc+, Prefibin 2 mg Sublingual Tablets. http://www.medicines.org.uk/EMC/medicine/25762/SPC/ Prefibin+2+mg+Sublingual+Tablets/.

79. A. Risedronate

Risedronate is a bisphosphonate salt, and the class is thought to have very poor bioavailability because of the formation of insoluble calcium salts when they are administered orally. Risedronate for instance has a bioavailability of only 0.63%, and this is diminished further when the agent is administered with food. For this reason, bisphosphonate administration is recommended first thing in the morning, on an empty stomach, with a glass of water. Patients are also recommended to remain upright for a period of time after taking the preparation. Bisphosphonates are associated with an increased risk of oesophagitis and oesophageal ulceration, although recent evidence suggests that this is not linked to increased risk of malignancy. Because of poor bioavailability, intermittent i.v. bisphosphonate preparations have been extensively developed. Actonel prescribing information, http://www.medicines.org.uk/ emc/medicine/11591.

80. B. Slow acetylation

Metabolism of isoniazid has acetylation as a key step. Polymorphism exists with respect to acetylation across the human population; in patients who are slow acetylators, isoniazid toxicity is increased because of accumulation. This may contribute to increased risk of hepatitis, and may also lead to increased risk of sideroblastic anaemia because of pyridoxine deficiency, due to accumulation of isoniazid. The elderly or those with evidence of malnutrition are usually supplemented with pyridoxine during therapy. With respect to hepatitis, therapy should be discontinued immediately, and careful consideration needs to be given as to whether it should be restarted or not, after LFTs have returned to normal.

emc+, Rifampicin: pharmacokinetic properties. http://www.medicines.org.uk/emc/medicine/8467#PHARMACOKINETIC_PROPS.

81. D. Cranberry juice

Increasing consumption of cranberry juice in the UK led to a number of yellow card reports about raised INR. Cranberry juice is a CYP450 enzyme inhibitor which leads to decreased warfarin metabolism and hence raised INR. Grapefruit juice is a specific 3A4 inhibitor and caution is advised about consumption in conjunction with statin use. For CYP450 interactions reviewed in detail see the link below.

Indiana University, Department of Medicine, Drug interactions. http://medicine.iupui.edu/clinpharm/ddis/.

82. C. CYP2D6

Three polymorphisms with respect to CYP2D6 activity are thought to exist: slow metabolizers, ultra fast metabolizers, and intermediate metabolizers, which lie between the two. The clinical significance of these polymorphisms is that in those who are ultra fast metabolizers, drug dosage may need to be increased if the agent administered undergoes significant 2D6 metabolism, and in those who are slow metabolizers, dose reduction may be required. In this case, metoprolol is metabolized by 2D6, and the clinical picture here of hypotension and bradycardia suggests that the patient is a slow metabolizer. He will either require dose reduction of his metoprolol or an alternative agent. The majority of beta-blockers are metabolized by 2D6, and as such an alternative such as a non-dihydropyridine calcium antagonist may be a better choice in this patient. Other drugs metabolized by 2D6 include a large number of anti-depressants and anti-psychotics.

Ingelman-Sundberg M, Genetic polymorphisms of cytochrome P450 2D6 (CYP2D6): clinical consequences, evolutionary aspects and functional diversity. http://www.nature.com/tpj/journal/v5/n1/full/6500285a.html.

83. D. Allopurinol

Allopurinol leads to accumulation of 6-mercaptopurine when it is co-prescribed with azathioprine, because xanthine oxidase is responsible for the metabolism and inactivation of 6-mercaptopurine. For this reason it is not recommended for the treatment of gout in patients taking azathioprine for chronic immunosuppression. Alternatives include colchicine, which can be dosed acutely up to 3 mg/day, and then the dosage reduced if chronic therapy is required. Prednisolone may also be used short term to overcome an acute attack of gout. Non-steroidals would usually not be recommended because of any risks to the renal transplant.

Drugs.com, Azathioprine. http://www.drugs.com/pro/azathioprine.html.

84. C. Give high flow oxygen and 0.5 ml 1:1000 adrenaline IM

This is a case of anaphylaxis related to penicillin. Anaphylaxis may occur in response to insect bites, food/food additives, and medication (antibiotics, blood products including IVIg, NSAIDs, and vaccinations). Initial management should be to establish an airway and give high flow oxygen. If there is refractory hypoxia, intubate and ventilate. Adrenaline should be given intramuscularly initially (dose 0.5 mg). Give IV hydrocortisone 200 mg, chlorpheniramine 10–20 mg, nebulizers, and fluid challenge as required. The rash that occurs with amoxicillin and Epstein–Barr virus is not associated with features of shock.

Simons FE, Anaphylaxis, *Journal of Allergy and Clinical Immunology* 2010;125(2, Suppl 2):S161–181.

85. C. Cystoscopy

Cyclophosphamide exposure increases the risk of bladder cancer. The risk increases with the cumulative dose of cyclophosphamide. Renal biopsy is not indicated as there is no evidence of active renal vasculitis—normal inflammatory markers, stable creatinine. The lack of abdominal pain makes urolithiasis unlikely. CT renal angiogram is used to investigate renal artery stenosis. This condition presents with hypertension, renal failure, flash pulmonary oedema, and does not associate with haematuria. Renal tract TB is unlikely in the absence of proteinuria.

Lapraik C et al., BSR and BHPR guidelines for the management of adults with ANCA associated vasculitis, *Rheumatology* 2007;46:1–11. http://www.rheumatology.org.uk/includes/documents/cm_docs/2009/m/management_of_adults_with_anca_associated_vasculitis.pdf.

86. B. Increased sodium in the distal segment of the distal tubule

Blockade of the thiazide-sensitive sodium chloride transporter in the proximal section of the distal convoluted tubule leads to increased delivery of sodium to the aldosterone-sensitive sodium, potassium, and hydrogen ion exchange pump in the distal portion of the distal tubule. This leads to increased potassium and hydrogen ion loss into urine and consequent hypokalaemia and increased serum bicarbonate. Thiazides also lead to conservation of calcium, which can be problematic in cases of dehydration in conjunction with continued diuretic use. Additionally, they are associated with a deterioration in glucose tolerance.

emc+, Natrilix: undesirable effects. http://www.medicines.org.uk/emc/medicine/1945/SPC/Natrilix/#UNDESIRABLE_EFFECTS.

87. B. Co-enzyme Q10 supplements

Ciprofloxacin, fluconazole, and metronidazole all inhibit the hepatic metabolism of warfarin and thus will cause an increased anti-coagulant effect of the same dose of warfarin. Acute alcohol consumption also causes hepatic enzyme inhibition and will increase the INR (chronic alcohol consumption on the other hand is an enzyme inducer and will reduce the anti-coagulant effect of warfarin). Co-enzyme Q10 is similar to vitamin K and reduces warfarin's anti-coagulant effect (warfarin exerts its anti-coagulant effect through inhibition of the synthesis of vitamin K-dependent clotting factors).

Richards D et al., *Oxford Handbook of Practical Drug Therapy*, Second Edition, Oxford University Press, 2011, Chapter 2, Cardiovascular system, Anticoagulants.

88. C. Endothelin A and B receptor antagonist

Endothelin is a key mediator which leads to the development and worsening of pulmonary hypertension, and endothelin receptor antagonists now form a backbone of medical therapy. Endothelin A receptors are predominantly involved in vasoconstriction, and endothelin B receptors lead to increased production of nitric oxide and prostacyclin, both vasodilators. Bosentan is a non-selective A and B receptor antagonist, ambrisentan is a selective A receptor antagonist. PDE-5 inhibitors also lead to a reduction in pulmonary hypertension.

emc+, Ambrisentan: pharmacodynamic properties. http://www.medicines.org.uk/emc/medicine/20848/SPC/Volibris/#PHARMACODYNAMIC_PROPS.

89. B. Glucagon

Glucagon stimulates production of cAMP by adenyl cyclase, but not via the beta-adrenergic pathways which normally provide sympathetic stimulation to the heart. In turn, cAMP increases heart rate and force of contraction. As such, it is the first-line treatment for management of beta-blocker overdose. Due to the short half-life of glucagon, intravenous infusion is typically required.

White CM, A review of potential cardiovascular uses of intravenous glucagon administration, *Journal of Clinical Pharmacology* 1999;39(5):442–447.

90. B. Atenolol

All except atenolol may increase the plasma concentration of digoxin, by displacement of digoxin from plasma binding sites or reducing clearance. Initiation of these drugs may require monitoring or adjustment of digoxin dosing. Symptoms of digoxin toxicity include nausea/vomiting, anorexia, diarrhoea, visual disturbance (xanthopsia), and confusion.

Rang HP, Dale MM, *Pharmacology*, Churchill Livingstone, 2007.

91. C. Ciprofloxacin

Both ciprofloxacin and clarithromycin are significant CYP450 inhibitors (predominantly 1A2 for ciprofloxacin and 3A4 for clarithromycin). This leads to an elevation in levels of theophylline which leads to tachycardia, nausea, and vomiting. In patients taking theophylline, physicians should be aware of the interaction and consider other options such as amoxicillin or doxycycline, or reduce the theophylline at the same time as starting the macrolide or ciprofloxacin. Azithromycin is a much weaker inhibitor of 3A4 than the other macrolides.

emc+, Uniphyllin Continus tablets. http://www.medicines.org.uk/emc/medicine/1233/SPC/Uniphyllin+Continus+tablets/.

92. E. Verapamil

Beta-blockers are not indicated in the treatment of cocaine overdose as they may exacerbate coronary artery spasm and lead to chest pain and possible infarction. The treatment of choice therefore to control an episode of paroxysmal SVT in this situation is a rate-limiting calcium antagonist such as verapamil or diltiazem. Ventricular arrhythmias are managed with sodium bicarbonate, with cautious use of lignocaine if the VT fails to resolve.

Ramrakha P et al., *Oxford Handbook of Acute Medicine*, Third Edition, Oxford University Press, 2010.

93. C. Intravenous magnesium sulphate

A Cochrane review has concluded that the treatment with the best evidence when the response to nebulizers and IV steroids is poor, is IV magnesium. Both IV aminophilline and IV salbutamol are associated with increased risk of rhythm disturbance and their therapeutic effect is only marginally superior to inhaled beta agonists. It is of course appropriate to assess the patient for an ITU admission. The following criteria help to decide the appropriateness of ITU care: hypoxia (PaO$_2$ <8 kPa (60 mmHg) despite FiO$_2$ of 60%; rising PaCO$_2$ or PaCO$_2$>6 kPa (45 mmHg); exhaustion, drowsiness, or coma; respiratory arrest; failure to improve despite adequate therapy.

Ramrakha P et al., *Oxford Handbook of Acute Medicine*, Third Edition, Oxford University Press, 2010.

94. A. Decreased phenytoin protein binding

Under normal conditions, phenytoin is highly protein bound. In conditions of renal failure however, the percentage of bound versus free phenytoin changes, so that more phenytoin is present in the unbound state. The assay for phenytoin levels however measures both the bound and the unbound component; this means that levels may appear to be in the normal range, but the patient still suffers symptoms of phenytoin toxicity. Phenytoin toxicity may also be precipitated by co-prescription of aspirin, which also increases the unbound portion of phenytoin.

Phenytoin summary of product characteristics. http://www.medicines.org.uk/emc/medicine/13289.

95. C. Intubation and ventilation

This patient has symptoms of a significant overdose of benzodiazepines. As such they are at risk from a compromised airway and require intervention. Whilst flumazenil is a benzodiazepine receptor antagonist, it is not recommended in the guidelines for treatment of benzodiazepine overdose because in patients habituated to use of the class, rapid reversal may precipitate seizures. For this reason, management involves airway protection until the sedative effects of the overdose have begun to resolve. Of course, naloxone is the reversal agent for opiate overdose, and glucagon for overdose of beta-blockers. Adrenalin is clearly not indicated in this situation.

emc+, Diazepam Tablets BP 10mg. http://www.medicines.org.uk/EMC/medicine/24401/SPC.

96. B. Feelings of depersonalization are seen

SSRI withdrawal is unpredictable, symptoms may last around a week in some patients, whilst in others they are still suffering months later. Nausea, vomiting, headaches, and insomnia are most commonly seen, and patients may complain of feelings of depersonalization. In fact, fluoxetine is less likely than other SSRIs to be associated with discontinuation syndrome. Problems can be avoided by gradual down-titration of the SSRI dose.

emc+, Prozac 20mg hard capsules, and 20mg per 5ml oral liquid. http://www.medicines.org.uk/emc/medicine/504/SPC/Prozac+20mg+hard+capsules,+and+20mg+per+5ml+oral+liquid/.

97. D. Intubation and ventilation

Introduction of flumazenil, the benzodiazepine antagonist, may precipitate severe agitation and fitting in a patient who is a habitual user of benzodiazepines. As this patient is known to use diazepam, there is a significant risk therefore to the use of flumazenil. As such, the most appropriate therapy here is intubation and ventilation, to allow for the effects of the alcohol and benzodiazepines to resolve. Without intubation the patient is at severe risk of aspiration.

Ramrakha P et al., *Oxford Handbook of Acute Medicine*, Third Edition, Oxford University Press, 2010.

98. E. Ketoprofen

Several reviews have taken place with respect to GI adverse events associated with NSAID use; azapropazone is associated with the highest risk, piroxicam and ketoprofen the next highest, diclofenac and naproxen intermediate risk, and ibuprofen has the least risk of GI adverse events. It is important to consider the lowest effective dose of therapy because of the risk of GI adverse events, and consider protection with a proton pump inhibitor such as omeprazole. In practice there is little difference between the SR and IR diclofenac and the risk of GI ulceration.

Russell RI, Non-steroidal anti-inflammatory drugs and gastrointestinal damage—problems and solutions, 2001;77:82–88 doi:10.1136/pmj.77.904.82.

99. D. It binds to penicillin binding protein

Carbapenems, of which imipenem is a member, bind to penicillin binding proteins. They are used to treat a variety of infections including generalized bacteraemia, pneumonia, intra-abdominal infections, obstetric and gynaecological infections, complicated urinary tract infections, and soft tissue and bone infections. It has poor oral bioavailability, is renally excreted, and therefore dose reduction is needed in renal failure, and it penetrates inflamed meninges. Resistance comes from penicillin binding protein mutations, reduced outer membrane permeability, and production of beta lactamases.

Torok E et al., *Oxford Handbook of Infectious Diseases and Microbiology*, Oxford University Press, 2009, Chapter 2, Antimicrobials, Carbapenems.

100. C. Metronidazole

The most likely diagnosis here is one of bacterial vaginosis. Caused by an overgrowth of mixed anaerobes such as Gardnerella and Mycoplasma, it results in secretion of amines in vaginal fluid, leading to the fishy odour. Clue cells are seen on microscopy, and vaginal pH is elevated at above 5.5. Metronidazole is the treatment of choice, either given as a single 2 g dose or as a course over 5 days. Clindamycin cream may also be of value.

Collins S et al., *Oxford Handbook of Obstetrics and Gynaecology*, Second Edition, Oxford University Press, 2008, Chapter 16, Genital tract infections, and pelvic pain, Bacterial vaginosis (BV). Arulkumaran S et al., *Oxford Handbook of Obstetrics and Gynaecology*, Second Edition, Oxford University Press, 2009.

101. B. H1 receptor antagonism

Cyclizine is a histamine H1 receptor antagonist, and as such is without the side effects associated with dopamine receptor antagonism such as acute dystonia and tardive dyskinesia. As such, it may be used in populations where metaclopramide and stemetil are relatively contraindicated, such as young women. Ondansetron is one of the family of 5-HT3 receptor antagonists, centrally acting anti-emetics, particularly useful in the management of chemotherapy-related nausea.

emc+, Valoid Tablets. http://www.medicines.org.uk/emc/medicine/14672.

102. A. Ethambutol

Standard short-course therapy for tuberculosis susceptible to the commonly used antimycobacterials consists of two months of therapy with the combination of isoniazid, rifampicin, pyrazinamide, and ethambutol. Treatment is then continued for a further four months with the reduced combination of isoniazid and rifampicin. Drug resistance is becoming increasingly common and greatly complicates therapy, particularly in cases of multi-drug resistant and extremely drug resistant tuberculosis. While drug therapy for tuberculosis is generally well tolerated, there are a number of important side effects and treatment should be monitored by a physician with experience in tuberculosis. While safety in pregnancy has not been rigorously established (and high doses of rifampicin were associated with teratogenicity in animal models), expert opinion and published guidelines suggest that pregnant women with symptomatic tuberculosis should be treated on the basis that the benefits outweigh the risks. The important

Table 4.2 Important adverse effects of TB therapy

Drug	Side effects
Isoniazid	Hepatotoxicity, gastrointestinal upset, peripheral neuropathy which can be prevented by co-administration of pyridoxine (vitamin B6), pancreatitis and psychiatric disorders
Rifampicin	Hepatotoxicity, gastrointestinal upset, orange discolouration of urine and other body fluids, influenza-like symptoms, acute rental impairment
Pyrazinamide	Hepatotoxicity, gastrointestinal upset, arthralgia, thrombocytopaenia
Ethambutol	Optic neuritis, red/green colour blindness

side effects of drugs commonly used in the management of TB are outlined in the table. As will be evident from Table 4.1, ethambutol is not associated with hepatotoxicity but can be associated with visual disturbance, and baseline visual acuity should be recorded for all patients prior to treatment with this drug. Patients should be warned to seek advice if they notice any visual symptoms while on therapy.

NICE guidelines [CG33], Tuberculosis: clinical diagnosis and management of tuberculosis, and measures for its prevention and control. https://www.nice.org.uk/guidance/cg33.

103. A. The lowest dose of NSAID to control symptoms should be used

When a patient is already using low-dose aspirin, NICE CG79 does not recommend concomitant prescription of NSAIDs. Instead, they recommend maximizing other pain-relieving medication ahead of adding an NSAID. In this case, regularizing use of paracetamol, then adding an opiate such as codeine would be initial steps, before considering an NSAID. If an NSAID is considered, then it should be started at the lowest appropriate dose, with addition of a PPI such as omeprazole for gastroprotection.

NICE guidelines [CG79], Rheumatoid arthritis in adults: management. https://www.nice.org.uk/guidance/CG79.

104. E. QT prolongation

Nucleoside reverse transcriptase inhibitors (NRTIs) are used in the management of HIV and hepatitis B infection. They inhibit the formation of DNA by reverse transcriptase and so inhibit viral replication. However, NRTIs also inhibit the transcription of human DNA, particularly mitochondrial DNA. This can lead to progressive mitochondrial dysfunction in patients treated with NRTIs. This can lead to myopathy, lactic actidosis, and lipodystrophy (alteration of the deposition of lipid tissue with loss of adiposity over the face, arms, and legs and accumulation of central adiposity with frequent appearance of a 'buffalo hump'). Zidovudine is strongly associated with the development of macrocytosis and is a not infrequent cause of anaemia and other haematological abnormalities. One NRTI (tenofovir) has been associated with renal tubular dysfunction and the development of associated calcium wasting with osteomalacia. QT prolongation is not a feature of NRTI therapy.

NAM aidsmap, HIV basics. http://www.aidsmap.com/hiv-basics.

105. A. Inhibitor of ErbB1 and ErbB2 receptors

Lapatanib is an inhibitor of the kinase domains of ErbB1 and ErbB2 (also known as EGFR and HER-2 receptors). It has been evaluated in a number of models and in cell lines which have been conditioned with trastuzumab, where it still appears to retain activity. In human clinical trials it has shown a prolongation of median time to progression, when added to capecitabine, versus capecitabine alone. Like trastuzumab, evaluation of left ventricular ejection fraction is necessary prior to commencing treatment. Other expected side effects include diarrhoea and liver function test abnormalities. Rarely, pulmonary toxicity has also been reported.

emc+, Lapatinib: pharmacodynamics properties. http://www.medicines.org.uk/emc/medicine/20929/SPC/Tyverb/#PHARMACODYNAMIC_PROPS.

106. C. She should stop methotrexate at least three months prior to trying for a baby

Methotrexate is a dihydrofolate reductase inhibitor, used in the treatment of a large range of autoimmune conditions and cancers. It is also teratogenic, and at high doses can cause craniofacial and limb defects as well as central nervous system abnormalities such as hydrocephaly. At lower doses such as those used for rheumatic disease, there is likely to be an increased chance of abortion. The BNF guidelines for this drug during pregnancy state: 'Avoid (teratogenic; fertility may be reduced during therapy but this may be reversible); effective contraception required during and for at least 3 months after treatment in women AND men.' It is therefore important to discuss plans for a family with both men and women in whom you are considering use of this drug.

In terms of medication that may be used, hydroxychloroquine and sulfasalazine pose minimal risk and these are the drugs of choice during pregnancy. If additional medication is required, then medications such as steroids, azathioprine, and TNF-alpha antagonists may be used selectively. They are usually considered when the benefits outweigh any potential risks. Medications that should be avoided altogether include methotrexate, leflunomide, cyclophosphamide, and mycophenolate mofetil. These are known to have the potential to cause harm. The United States Food and Drug Administration is a good source of information as it categorizes drugs according to risk in pregnancy.

Janssen NM et al., The effects of immunosuppressive and anti-inflammatory medications on fertility, pregnancy, and lactation, *Archives of Internal Medicine* 2000;160:610–619.

107. E. Metformin

This patient is overweight and has gestational diabetes. She has been unable to manage her blood glucose control successfully with diet and exercise and therefore requires an intervention. Both glibenclamide and metformin now have evidence in the treatment of gestational diabetes mellitus, but out of the two, glibenclamide is likely to cause weight gain and as such is not the best option. Metformin has been validated in a large study with insulin rescue, and has been shown to be associated with increased patient treatment satisfaction and no detrimental impact on neonatal outcomes.

Nice guidelines [CG64], Diabetes in pregnancy: management of diabetes and its complications from pre-conception to the postnatal period. http://www.nice.org.uk/Guidance/CG63.

108. A. Type 1

The immediate nature of the reaction, and the patch testing favour a type 1 hypersensitivity reaction here. RAST testing is an alternative to patch testing, and it is important to investigate reactions like this because of the use of egg products in the preparation of vaccines and a number of excipients and preservatives that may be added in their preparation.

Wilkins R et al., *Oxford Handbook of Medical Sciences*, Second Edition, Oxford University Press, 2011, Chapter 12, Infection and immunity, Hypersensitivity.

109. C. Bisoprolol

Amongst cardiovascular agents, ACE inhibitors, angiotensin receptor blockers, calcium channel blockers, and beta-blockers are particularly recognized to be associated with the development of psoriasis. Withdrawal of the potential offending agent is the management of choice. Other agents known to be associated with psoriasis include antimalarials, bupropion, carbamazepine, interferon (IFN) alfa, lithium, metformin, NSAIDs, terbinafine, tetracyclines, valproate sodium, and venlafaxine.

Collier J et al., *Oxford Handbook of Clinical Specialities*, Eighth Edition, Oxford University Press, 2009, Chapter 8, Dermatology, Psoriasis.

110. A. Absorption

The rate of absorption of a particular agent is likely to have the biggest impact with respect to t-max, the time taken after administration for maximal plasma concentration to be reached. Drugs that are predominantly absorbed in the distal small bowel, for example, are likely to have a significantly longer t-max than those that are absorbed in the stomach or the proximal part of the small bowel. Small bowel villi increase the surface area greatly with respect to absorption, and hence the small bowel is the site of absorption of most oral drugs. Some highly polar compounds such as digoxin may be easily absorbed via membrane ion channels. Other large molecules such as aminoglycoside antibiotics cannot be delivered orally because they have little or no absorption because of their molecular size.

Le J, Drug absorbtion, Merck manual. http://www.merck.com/mmpe/sec20/ch303/ch303b.html.

111. E. The drug is transported bound to plasma proteins

Metformin, a biguanide oral hypoglycaemic agent, is used as first-line drug treatment for overweight patients with type 2 diabetes. It is particularly suitable for this population as it improves insulin sensitivity and suppresses appetite. This leads to an improvement in glycaemic control, comparable to that seen with sulphonylurea use, but with significantly less weight gain. The antihyperglycaemic effect of metformin is achieved through various mechanisms including suppression of hepatic glucose output and increase in (insulin-mediated) glucose disposal. The most serious adverse effects of metformin is lactic acidosis and a previous biguanide (phenformin) was withdrawn for this association. Although serious, the risk of this lactic acidosis with metformin therapy is low, particularly when prescribing guidelines and contraindications are adhered to. Current NICE guidance states that the dose of metformin should be reviewed when creatinine exceeds 130 µmol/l (eGFR <45) and stopped when creatinine exceeds 150 µmol/l (or eGFR <30). In terms of pharmacokinetics, metformin is rapidly distributed following gastrointestinal absorption but does not bind to plasma proteins. It has a bioavailability of 40–60% following oral ingestion and an onset of action within days. The drug does not undergo liver metabolism and there are no known metabolites. It is renally excreted (90% unchanged) and has a plasma half-life of 4–9 hours.

NICE guidelines [CG87], Type 2 diabetes: the management of type 2 diabetes. https://www.nice.org.uk/guidance/cg87.

112. B. Four hours

The half-life is calculated from the time when maximal concentration is reached. From two hours after administration (maximal concentration point) to four hours, the concentration reduces by 25%; this means that it is likely to reduce by 50% at the six-hour time point. Essentially this means that the half-life of the new agent is four hours, the time taken for concentration to fall to 50% of the maximum. A number of things can affect half-life. These include the polarity of the compound, if it is highly water soluble, or predominantly lipophilic. Also if it undergoes extensive hepatic metabolism or if it is mainly excreted by the kidneys. Route of metabolism/excretion needs to be taken into account when assessing where dose frequency or level may need to be altered according to pre-existing disease or concomitant medications.

Oh P, Clinical pharmacology. http://www.ucl.ac.uk/anaesthesia/education/Pharmacology.

113. B. Use emollients

The likely diagnosis is asteatotic eczema which is a common problem and will improve with emollients. The other options may be appropriate when the patient's condition does not respond to emollients.

Patient, Asteatotic Eczema (Eczema Craquelé). http://www.patient.co.uk/doctor/Asteatotic-Eczema-(Eczema-Craquele).htm.

114. B. Dry cough

Ramipril is a commonly used anti-hypertensive. Some patients get a dry cough as a side effect of the angiotensin converting enzyme inhibitor (ACEI). ACEIs lead to reduced breakdown of bradykinin, the cause of the cough. Impotence is most commonly reported in patients treated with thiazides or beta-blockers. Angioedema is thankfully only rarely seen in patients treated with ACE inhibitors. Regular monitoring of renal function is indicated after commencement of therapy as in the case of underlying renal artery stenosis, a rapid deterioration in renal function may be seen. Gout is seen most commonly in patients treated with thiazides.

Longmore M et al., *Oxford Handbook of Clinical Medicine*, Eighth Edition, Oxford University Press, 2010, Chapter 3, Cardiovascular medicine, Heart failure—Management.

115. E. Digoxin

First-pass metabolism is the metabolism of an agent by the liver on its first pass through the organ after being absorbed from the intestine and carried via the hepatic portal vein. Unless the first-pass metabolism results in conversion of a prodrug to an active metabolite, it can limit the systemic effectiveness of an agent considerably. Agents that are known to have a high degree of first-pass metabolism include propranolol, hydralazine, levodopa, and nitrates. Digoxin has a particularly low first-pass metabolism, which may be related to its high degree of water solubility. Other drugs that have a low first-pass metabolism include the benzodiazepines (which are highly distributed into peripheral tissues), phenytoin, and warfarin. High first-pass metabolism can be overcome via alternative methods of delivery, such as IV delivery, intranasal, transpulmonary, or subcutaneous routes. It can also be overcome by delivering the agent as a prodrug, which is then metabolized by the liver to produce an active. An example here is enalapril, which undergoes relatively high hepatic first-pass metabolism. This has a low impact on effectiveness, however, as enalapril is metabolized in vivo by esterases to form enalaprilat, the main active form.

Oh P, Clinical pharmacology. http://www.ucl.ac.uk/anaesthesia/education/Pharmacology.

116. B. Ciprofloxacin

Theophylline is metabolized by CYP 1A2, and the symptoms given here are consistent with a diagnosis of theophylline toxicity. Out of the antibiotics listed, ciprofloxacin is an inhibitor of the 1A2 isoenzyme, hence this is the most likely antibiotic that he was prescribed. Macrolide antibiotics are inhibitors of CYP 3A4, but azithromycin is not considered a significant 3A4 inhibitor. Penicillins do not have a significant interaction with theophylline, hence both amoxicillin and co-amoxiclav would be reasonable options with respect to treating an upper respiratory tract infection in this patient.

emc+, Slo-Phyllin 60mg, 125mg, 250mg, Capsules. http://www.medicines.org.uk/emc/medicine/1047.

117. B. Grapefruit juice

Simvastatin is metabolized by CYP 3A4. Inhibitors of CYP 3A4 include macrolide antibiotics and grapefruit juice. Rifampicin is a potent cytochrome P450 enzyme inducer, which means that co-prescription with statins is likely to increase their metabolism and decrease their effect. The data sheet for simvastatin is very clear, that use with grapefruit juice is prohibited. Across the range of statins the risk of myopathy appears similar apart from cerivastatin where a higher rate of myopathy was seen (5–10 times the rate of currently available statins), and it was withdrawn after over 400 cases of rhabdomyolysis. This led to particular concern about co-prescription of statins with fibrates, but recent trial evidence has largely allayed fears about a significant increase in myopathy events.

Indiana University, Department of Medicine, Clinical Pharmacology, Drug Interactions: defining genetic influences on pharmacologic responses. http://medicine.iupui.edu/clinpharm/ddis/.

118. C. Rifampicin

Rifampicin is a hepatic enzyme inducer, and causes the liver enzymes that metabolize warfarin to increase their productivity. This causes increased warfarin breakdown and a reduction in INR. Ciprofloxacin, omeprazole, erythromycin, and allopurinol are hepatic enzyme inhibitors. They can therefore reduce the rate of warfarin metabolism and increase the INR. Warfarin is metabolized primarily by cytochrome p450 enzymes in the liver. These can be affected by a large number of other medications which can induce or inhibit these enzymes. This can therefore alter the INR. In this case, it is particularly important to maintain a therapeutic INR as the patient has a high-risk metallic valve. In cases such as this, it is useful to be aware of common medications that affect hepatic enzymes so that the INR can be monitored more frequently or an alternative medication can be used. Common P450 enzyme inducers include: rifampicin, anticonvulsants—phenytoin and carbamezapine, chronic alcohol use. Common p450 enzyme inhibitors include: omeprazole, cimetidine, antibiotics—ciprofloxacin, erythromycin, sulfonamides, allopurinol, and acute alcohol intoxication. It is important to think about the effects of new medication on current drugs. If in doubt, check the BNF.

BNF Appendix 1: section on phamacokinetic interactions. https://www.evidence.nhs.uk/formulary/bnf/current/a1-interactions/pharmacokinetic-interactions.

119. C. Bendroflumethiazide

Lithium is renally excreted so toxicity can be a problem in patients with impaired renal function, or in patients who are commenced on medications that disturb renal function. Thiazide diuretics such as bendroflumethiazide are commonly implicated in the development of lithium toxicity. Thiazides act by decreasing sodium ion resorption in the kidney and therefore increasing potassium excretion. It is thought that lithium ions in the renal filtrate may be exchanged with potassium ions as they are excreted, thus leading to retention of lithium and the risk of toxicity. Medications such as loop diuretics, non-steroidal anti-inflammatories, and angiotensin converting enzyme inhibitors may also lead to increased serum levels of lithium due to their relative nephrotoxic effects. Calcium channel blockers, such as amlodipine, can also be associated with lithium toxicity, but less frequently when compared to bendroflumethiazide. The other medications listed do not affect lithium levels.

Nicholson J, Fitzmaurice B, Monitoring patients on lithium—a good practice guideline, *Psychiatrist* 2002;26:348–351. http://pb.rcpsych.org/cgi/content/full/26/9/348.

120. D. Atorvastatin

Drug-induced liver injury is common and may be considered in terms of hepatocellular, cholestatic, fibrotic, vascular, and granulomatous injury. Some drugs may produce jaundice by inducing haemolysis (e.g. dapsone). Elevation of the alkaline phosphatase in excess of hepatic transaminases indicates a cholestatic pattern of injury/jaundice. Co-amoxiclav, nitrofurantoin, combined oral contraceptives, and sulphonylureas all cause cholestatic injury. In contrast, statins cause a hepatocellular pattern of injury (transaminases elevated in excess of alkaline phosphatase).

Longmore M et al., *Oxford Handbook of Clinical Medicine*, Eighth Edition, Oxford University Press, 2010, Chapter 6, Gastroenterology, Jaundice.

121. E. Enoxaparin

Hyperkalaemia is most likely to be due to enoxaparin.

Amlodipine and chlordiazepoxide are not associated with hyperkalaemia. Ibuprofen, like other non-steroidal anti-inflammatory drugs, can be nephrotoxic and can induce hyperkalaemia by causing renal impairment. The normal urea and creatinine rule this out in this case.

For a review of hyperkalaemia including causes: http://emedicine.medscape.com/article/240903-overview.

122. A. Hepatic impairment

Gentamicin is an aminoglycoside that is bactericidal and is a protein synthesis inhibitor. Aminoglycosides are often used to treat infections caused by Gram-negative organisms. They are not absorbed from the gut so must be administered intravenously. Side effects include renal impairment, which is a significant risk, so drug levels must be carefully monitored. Ototoxicity is also a recognized complication of gentamicin therapy. Stomatitis, hypomagnesaemia, nausea, vomiting, rash, and neuromuscular transmission impairment have also been observed. Aminoglycosides are renally as opposed to hepatically excreted; therefore, hepatic impairment is not a recognized side effect of gentamicin therapy.

British National Formulary, Edition 60, September 2010, BMJ Group, Online edition. https://www.evidence.nhs.uk/formulary/bnf/current/5-infections/51-antibacterial-drugs/514-aminoglycosides/gentamicin.

123. B. Phase 2

Phase 1 studies are usually conducted in healthy volunteers, unless the therapy being trialled is significantly toxic, in which case it is carried out in patients who have a particular disease (e.g. HIV, cancer indication, and some monoclonal antibody indications). Phase 2 studies look at surrogate markers, such as in the case of diabetes, short-term changes in HbA1c or fasting blood glucose, across a range of doses. The one that has the best efficacy/tolerability profile is then taken forward into a phase 3 study programme. Phase 4 studies test efficacy in a clinical setting. Health outcomes data may come from the phase 3 programme, or additionally from database studies in a real-life population, such as the GPRD database operated by the MHRA (UK medicines regulator).

Clinicaltrials.gov, Learn about clinical studies. http://clinicaltrials.gov/ct2/info/understand.

124. D. MHRA

With respect to safety, only the MHRA is able to make decisions about the safety of marketed medicinal products and their benefit risk. NICE is able to make decisions about the cost effectiveness of drugs, and local prescribing committees take decisions about access to medicines based on safety and cost effectiveness grounds. It is important not to confuse the roles and responsibilities of the various authorities in determining safety of and access to medicines. The Scottish Medicines Consortium makes similar rulings to NICE with respect to Scotland.

gov.uk, MHRA. http://www.mhra.gov.uk/index.htm.

125. E. Aspirin

The reader should familiarize themselves with the current guidelines for management of chronic atrial fibrillation and can refer to the RCP and NICE guidelines published. Digoxin is not appropriate for this patient as it is clear that his AF is rate-controlled. The patient does not require warfarinization due to his age and also lack of co-morbidities. Therefore aspirin is the correct anser as he is less than 65 years old with no previous history of a CVA or additional risk factors.

Atrial fibrillation: management

NICE guidelines [CG180] Published date: June 2014 https://www.nice.org.uk/guidance/cg180.

126. A. CTA (clinical trial application)

A range of information is required as part of the application, which includes pre-clinical data, clinical data in other indications, rationale for the new study, and design of the proposed clinical trial. Also important are the qualifications and training of investigators and their ability to conduct the study as proposed. There are a number of acronyms to do with clinical trials, these include the BLA (biological licence application), NDA (new drug application), and IND (investigational new drug application).

gov.uk, Clinical trials for medicines: apply for authorisation in the UK. http://www.mhra.gov.uk/Howweregulate/Medicines/Licensingofmedicines/Clinicaltrials/Clinicaltrialsformedicinalproducts/index.htm.

127. E. Sodium valproate

Sodium valproate and ethosuximide would normally be considered first-line anti-epileptics for absence seizures.

Manji H et al., *Oxford Handbook of Neurology*, Oxford University Press, 2006, Chapter 4, Neurological disorders.

128. E. Doxazosin and carbamazepine

Doxazosin and carbamazepine have no known significant interaction. Calcium salts may inhibit the absorption of levothyroxine, as indeed may iron. Preparations should be given at a different time of day. Concomitant methotrexate and trimethoprim use results in an increased risk of haematological toxicity and bone marrow suppression—likely due to folate antagonism. Simvastatin is metabolized by the cytochrome P450 isoenzyme CYP34A. Clarithromycin is a potent inhibitor of CYP34A and the resulting reduction in simvastatin metabolism can cause significantly raised levels and side effects such as myopathy or even rhabdomyolysis. Using omeprazole in conjunction with clopidogrel blocks the CYP450 2C19-mediated bio-activation of clopidogrel, reducing the cardioprotective benefit.

British National Formulary. http://bnf.org.

129. A. Inhibition of URAT-1

Losartan is an inhibitor of URAT-1, which in turn promotes excretion of uric acid. This accounts for the improvement in serum urate seen after starting the blood pressure therapy. Colchicine inhibits formation of intracellular microtubules, allopurinol is a xanthine oxidase inhibitor. Recombinate uricases are available to promote urate metabolism, and are used in prevention of acute urate nephropathy in patients undergoing chemotherapy.

Hamada T et al., Uricosuric action of losartan via the inhibition of urate transporter 1 (URAT 1) in hypertensive patients. *American Journal of Hypertension* 2008;21:1157–1162.

130. C. Metaclopramide

Metaclopramide is a D2 antagonist antiemetic, and as such is associated with acute dystonia (the presentation here) and tardive dyskinesia. Acute dystonia occurs more frequently in young women and as such is best avoided in this situation. Whilst domperidone is also a dopamine antagonist, it is not usually associated with acute dystonia. Cyclizine and promethazine are anti-histamine anti-emetics and are reasonable options in this population, as is ondansetron which works through the 5-HT system.

Edwards M, Quinn N, Bhatia K, *Oxford Specialist Handbook of Parkinson's Disease and Other Movement Disorders,* Oxford University Press, 2008, Chapter 10, Drug-induced movement disorders.

131. E. Supportive therapy only

In most cases, mild drowsiness is the major consequence of sodium valproate overdose. Hypotension, unconsciousness, seizures, coma, and respiratory failure are, however, reported at total doses above 5 g. Fatalities have been reported above 20 g total dose. Induced vomiting, gastric lavage, activated charcoal, and haemodialysis are not indicated in the management of valproate overdose. Depending on level of consciousness and blood pressure, respiratory and circulatory support may, however, be required.

Ramrakha P et al., *Oxford Handbook of Acute Medicine,* Third Edition, Oxford University Press, 2010.

132. A. Flumazenil

Flumazenil is useful for short-term reversal of benzodiazepine-mediated respiratory depression and decreased consciousness. It is not, however, recommended in patients who are habitual users of benzodiazepines, particularly in conjunction with tricyclic anti-depressants, as withdrawal can precipitate seizures. In this case, however, reversal will make the patient's airway significantly easier to manage. Glucagon is used in the treatment of beta-blocker overdose, naloxone in opiate overdose.

Wyatt JP et al., *Oxford Handbook of Emergency Medicine,* Fourth Edition, Oxford University Press, 2012.

133. B. It is likely to have a large volume of distribution

Drugs which are highly lipid soluble are rapidly redistributed to peripheral tissues and can cross the blood–brain barrier relatively easily, a prime example being the benzodiazepine class. This leads to a short half life as measured drug in plasma falls rapidly. Renal excretion occurs most efficiently for polar substances which are very water soluble. Hence this agent is likely to require metabolism by the liver prior to its excretion. Lipid soluble agents are poorly soluble in water and infusion solutions, and are usually injected as emulsions if IV delivery is required.

Tasker RC et al., *Oxford Handbook of Paediatrics,* Second Edition, Oxford University Press, 2013.

134. C. Haemodialysis

This patient has a very significant lithium overdose, and haemodialysis is recommended when the lithium level is >4 mmol/L. Whole bowel irrigation is only recommended where a slow-release lithium preparation has been taken. Activated charcoal does not absorb lithium, and gastric lavage is only useful in the first hour after overdose. Induced vomiting is not recommended in any circumstances.

Wyatt JP et al., *Oxford Handbook of Emergency Medicine*, Fourth Edition, Oxford University Press, 2012.

135. E. 100%

The dose of paraquat ingested is a good predictor of outcome, with death reported after only 10–15 mL of the 20% solution (3 g) of paraquat. Death is universal after ingestion of 50 mL (10 g). Plasma levels of paraquat >2 mg/L at four hours or 0.1 mg/L at 24 hours are associated with a poor prognosis. Activated charcoal may be given when patients present within one hour of paraquat ingestion. Haemodialysis is only considered where smaller amounts of paraquat are ingested, as haemodialysis is not very effective at removing it. A low WBC on admission carries a poor prognosis.

Ramrakha P et al., *Oxford Handbook of Acute Medicine*, Third Edition, Oxford University Press, 2010, Chapter 14, Drug overdoses.

136. B. High molecular weight

Solubility of oral preparations is influenced both by molecular weight and polarity. Drugs that are most easily absorbed tend to be more polar and of relatively low molecular weight, otherwise they might need to be administered as a suspension or as an oily solution. Twenty per cent renal excretion implies that the agent is likely to have no problem with administration in patients with moderate renal impairment, and may even be acceptable for use in those with severe renal impairment. CYP2C9 is responsible for the metabolism of warfarin, so an interaction study would be needed, but 2C9 metabolism does not preclude development in any way. A half life of nine hours is likely to mean once or twice daily dosing at steady state, acceptable for an anti-hypertensive.

Steddon S, et al., *Oxford Handbook of Nephrology and Hypertension*, Oxford University Press, 2006, Chapter 11, Pregnancy and the kidney.

137. E. Dabigatran 150 mg BD

Given frequent foreign travel, it is going to be difficult for this patient to be compliant with warfarin monitoring. In this situation NICE technology appraisal endorses dabigatran as an alternative option.

NICE (2012). Dabigatran etexilate for the prevention of stroke and systemic embolism in atrial fibrillation. http://publications.nice.org.uk/ dabigatran-etexilate-for-the-prevention-of-stroke-and-systemic-embolism-in-atrial-fibrillation-ta249.

138. B. Lamotrigine

Phenytoin and carbamazepine are P450 enzyme inducers and as such they reduce the effectiveness of the oral contraceptive pill, meaning this patient may run the risk of getting pregnant. In addition phenytoin may lead to gum hypertrophy. Sodium valproate is associated with weight gain and a PCOS-like syndrome in women. Retigabine is a treatment for partial epilepsy and is usually prescribed as an adjunct to other therapies. In general, sodium valproate is used as first-line therapy for generalized epilepsy as monotherapy. Where valproate is unsuitable, lamotrigine is the initial first option of choice. Levitiracetam, valproate, and lamotrigine are all used in combination for patients who continue to seizure. Partial seizures are managed first line with lamotrigine or carbamazepine.

emc+, Lamictal. http://www.medicines.org.uk/emc/medicine/4228/SPC/lamictal/.

INDEX

Escherichia coli 24*at*
ethambutol, adverse effects 190*a*, 206*at*
ethylene glycol poisoning 142*q*, 160*q*, 185*a*, 198*a*
extradural haematomas 18*qf*, 35*a*
ezetimibe
    adverse effects 196*a*
    mechanism of action 158*q*, 196*a*, 198*a*

F

Fabry's disease 115*a*
factor VII deficiency 57*a*
factor V Leiden mutation 49*q*, 64*a*
faecal calprotectin 187*a*
Fallot's tetralogy 125*a*
familial adenomatous polyposis 26*a*
familial cancers 6*q*, 25*a*–26*a*
fatigue 39*q*
febrile non-haemolytic transfusion reaction 60*a*
fenofibrate 154*q*–155*q*, 161*q*, 194*a*
FGFR3 gene mutations 26*a*
fibrates
    combination with statins 194*a*
    mechanism of action 154*q*–155*q*, 161*q*, 194*a*, 198*a*
first-pass metabolism 175*q*, 209*a*
fluconazole, drug interactions 190*a*
fludarabine 184*a*
flumazenil 200*a*, 204*a*, 213*a*
fluorouracil, mechanism of action 184*a*, 200*a*
fluoxetine, withdrawal of medication 169*q*, 204*a*
FMR-1 hypermethylation 7*q*, 26*a*
focal seizures, management 145*q*, 188*a*
fomepizole, mechanism of action 142*q*, 160*q*, 185*a*,
    197*a*–198*a*
fondaparinux 135*a*
fragile-X syndrome 26*a*, 33*a*
Friedreich's ataxia 25*a*
frontal lobe lesions 7*q*, 27*a*
fungal endocarditis 86*q*, 121*a*
furosemide
    mechanism of action 139*q*, 184*a*
    site of action 4*q*, 23*a*

G

gallstones 49*q*, 64*a*
gangliosides 32*a*
gemtuzomab 191*a*
genetic disorders 2*q*, 3*q*, 6*q*
    achondroplasia 7*q*, 26*a*
    autosomal recessive inheritance 2*q*, 3*q*
    Brugada syndrome 119*a*
    Carney syndrome 75*q*, 114*a*–115*a*
    cystic fibrosis 3*q*, 22*a*, 88*q*
Down's syndrome 33*a*, 120*a*
    Duchenne muscular dystrophy 21*a*
    Edward's syndrome 16*q*, 33*a*
    familial cancers 6*q*, 25*a*–26*a*
    FMR-1 hypermethylation 7*q*, 26*a*

Friedreich's ataxia 25*a*
haemochromatosis 7*q*, 21*a*, 26*a*–27*a*
haemophilia 38*q*, 56*a*
Huntington's disease 19*q*
Klinefelter syndrome 5*q*, 24*a*
Leber's optic neuropathy 16*q*
mitochondrial disorders 11*q*, 29*a*, 33*a*
retinoblastoma 15*q*
Stickler syndrome 21*a*
tuberous sclerosis 21*a*
Turner syndrome 1*q*, 4*q*, 20*a*, 23*a*
gentamicin, adverse effects 178*q*, 211*a*
gestational diabetes 173*q*, 207*a*
Gilbert's syndrome 64*a*
Glasgow Coma Scale (GCS) 19*q*, 35*a*
glitazone therapy
    adverse effects 154*q*, 193*a*
    mechanism of action 194*a*
glucagon, in beta-blocker overdose 203*a*
gluconeogenesis 23*a*
glucose 6 phosphate deficiency 48*q*, 63*a*
glucose levels, regulation of 23*a*
glucose phosphate isoenzyme BB (GPBB), levels after
        MI 113*a*
glycogenolysis 23*a*
goitre, amiodarone-induced thyroiditis 139*q*, 184*a*
Golgi apparatus 21*a*
Goodpasture's disease 188*a*
gout, alternatives to allopurinol 201*a*
graft versus host disease (GVHD), transfusion-mediated 60*a*
Gram-staining 4*q*, 6*q*, 24*at*, 25*a*
grapefruit juice, drug interactions 201*a*, 209*a*
gynaecomastia, drug-induced 108*q*, 162*q*, 199*a*

H

haematemesis 45*q*
haematuria, investigation of 166*q*, 202*a*
haemochromatosis 21*a*, 98*q*, 118*a*, 127*a*
    genetic defect 7*q*, 26*a*–27*a*
haemoglobin dissociation curve 5*q*, 24*a*
haemolysis, drug-induced 48*q*, 63*a*
haemolysis of blood samples, spurious hyperkalaemia 29*a*
haemophilia 33*a*
    genetic counselling 38*q*, 56*a*
Haemophilus influenzae 24*at*, 25*a*
haemorrhage
    epistaxis 51*q*
    haematemesis 45*q*
    intracranial 18*qf*, 34*a*–35*a*, 43*q*, 60*a*
half-life 174*q*, 208*a*
haloperidol, adverse effects 150*q*, 191*a*
head injuries 18*q*–19*q*, 34*a*–35*a*
heart failure 95*q*–96*q*, 136*a*
    acute management 94*q*, 111*q*, 125*a*
    aldosterone antagonists 108*q*, 134*a*–135*a*
    beta-blockers 118*a*, 132*a*, 135*a*
    cardiac resynchronization therapy 126*a*

sunitinib 191*a*
  adverse effects 188*a*
superficial temporal artery 35*a*
superior vena cava obstruction 53*q*, 67*a*
supraventricular tachycardia (SVT) 99*q*, 101*q*, 128*a*,
      129*a*–130*a*
  differentiation from VT 110*q*, 136*a*
  during pregnancy 100*q*, 129*a*
sympathetic nervous system, anatomy 34*a*
syphilis 144*q*, 187*a*

T

tacrolimus
  adverse effects 196*a*
  mechanism of action 186*a*
tamoxifen resistance 54*q*, 67*a*
tenofovir, adverse effects 206*a*
testicular cancer 55*q*, 68*a*
theophylline, drug interactions 176*q*, 198*a*, 203*a*, 209*a*
thiazides
  adverse effects 156*a*, 189*a*, 195*a*
  as cause of hypokalaemia 166*q*, 202*a*
  drug interactions 210*a*
thrombocytopenia
  after red cell transfusion 61*a*
  in pregnancy 38*q*, 57*a*
thrombotic thrombocytopenic purpura 47*q*, 62*a*–63*a*
thyroid disease, amiodarone-induced thyroiditis
      139*q*, 184*a*
tissue Doppler echocardiography 127*a*
T-max, influencing factors 174*q*, 208*a*
TMPT (thiopurine s-methyl transferase) activity 9*q*, 28*a*,
      187*a*
TORCH study 195*a*
torsades de pointes 130*a*
tranexamic acid, mechanism of action 51*q*, 65*a*
transfer factor 1*q*, 2*q*, 20*a*
  in asthma 21*a*
transfusion-dependent anaemia 60*a*
transfusion reactions 42*q*–43*q*, 46*q*
  febrile non-haemolytic 60*a*
  platelet transfusions 61*a*–62*a*
  rhesus incompatibility 59*a*
  transfusion-associated lung injury (TRALI) 59*a*, 61*a*
transverse sinus 35*a*
tricuspid regurgitation 98*q*, 127*a*–128*a*
troponin levels 113*a*
T-test 30*a*
tuberculosis (TB), treatment 205*a*
  adverse effects of 171*q*, 206*at*
tuberous sclerosis 21*a*
tumour lysis syndrome, prevention of 151*q*
tumour markers 2*q*, 21*a*
Turner syndrome 1*q*, 4*q*, 23*a*
  causes of death 20*a*
type I errors 30*a*
type II errors 11*q*, 30*a*

U

urate levels, effect of losartan 180*q*, 212*a*
uricosuric drugs 192*a*

V

vaccinations
  hypersensitivity reactions 207*a*
  during pregnancy 144*q*, 187*a*
vagal stimulation techniques 123*a*
  cautions 129*a*
vaginal discharge 171*q*, 205*a*
valproate see sodium valproate
valsartan, in heart failure 132*a*
venous thromboembolism
  deep venous thrombosis 49*q*, 52*q*, 63*a*–64*a*, 66*a*
  management in cancer patients 51*q*, 65*a*
  prophylaxis see anticoagulation
ventral root injuries 16*q*, 33*a*–34*a*
ventricular arrhythmia, management 72*q*, 73*q*, 113*a*
ventricular septal defect 124*a*–125*a*
  post-MI 135*a*
ventricular tachycardia 84*q*, 85*qf*, 113*a*, 114*a*, 119*a*–120*a*,
      189*a*
  in amitriptyline overdose 147*q*
  cocaine-induced 203*a*
  differentiation from SVT 110*q*, 136*a*
verapamil, drug interactions 186*a*
vincristine 184*a*
vitamin B_{12} deficiency 58*a*
vitamin K deficiency 57*a*
V_{max}, enzyme-catalysed reactions 13*q*–14*qf*, 31*a*

W

warfarin
  alternatives to 182*q*, 214*a*
  drug interactions 176*q*, 201*a*, 210*a*
  in factor V Leiden mutation 49*q*, 64*a*
  management of high INR 51*q*, 66*a*
  mechanism of action 57*a*, 65*a*
  potentiating factors 50*q*, 64*a*, 164*q*, 166*q*, 202*a*
  and pregnancy 59*a*
  subarachnoid haemorrhage management 43*q*, 60*a*
Wolf–Parkinson–White syndrome 77*qf*, 115*a*
working memory 36*a*

X

X-linked disorders 33*a*
  haemophilia 56*a*

Y

Y-linked disorders 33*a*

Z

zidovudine, adverse effects 206*a*
zomatriptan 194*a*
Z scores 30*a*